THE DIABETES REFERENCE BOOK

THE DIABETES REFERENCE BOOK

Direct and Clear Answers to Everyone's Questions

by
Peter H Sönksen, MD, FRCP
Professor of Endocrinology, St Thomas' Hospital Medical
School, and Honorary Consultant Physician, St Thomas'
Hospital, London

Charles Fox, BM, MRCP
Physician with Special Interest in Diabetes,
Northampton General Hospital
and
Sue Judd, SRN
Specialist Sister in Diabetes, St Thomas' Hospital, London

*Forewords by Doctor Arnold Bloom, Chairman, British
Diabetic Association and Sir Harry Secombe, CBE,
President of British Diabetic Association.*

Harper & Row, Publishers
London

Cambridge San Francisco
Mexico City São Paulo
New York Singapore
Philadelphia Sydney

First published 1985
Reprinted 1986

Harper & Row Ltd
28 Tavistock Street
London WC2E 7PN

British Library Cataloguing in Publication Data

Sönksen, P.H.
  The diabetes reference book.
  1. Diabetes
  I. Title   II. Fox, C.J.   III. Judd S.L.
  616.4'62   RC660

ISBN 0 06 318313 7

Typeset by Burns & Smith, Derby
Printed and bound by Butler & Tanner Ltd, Frome and London

NOTE: All information was correct at time of going to press.

Contents

Foreword

Diabetes is a life-long disorder, and the better it is managed, the better the outlook for a long and healthy life. But no one should be expected to follow a lot of restrictions and advice unless their purpose is fully understood. Questions keep cropping up — and here we have the answers, clearly expressed and sympathetic in approach. The book is written by three experts in the field with a wide knowledge, experience and understanding of the problems to be explained.

I am sure this book will be a friend and guide not only for those with diabetes but also for those who play a part in helping them at home.

Arnold Bloom
Chairman, British Diabetic Association

Foreword

Everyone knows the importance of education in our lives, but if you have diabetes, then learning certainly becomes a way of life.

As someone with diabetes, I realise the more I know about the condition and the way it affects me, the healthier I stay.

So I have no hesitation in commending this book, compiled by people whose active involvement with diabetes is an example to everyone.

Sir Harry Secombe, CBE

Acknowledgements

British Diabetic Association:
  Balance — Jenny Dyer, previous editor.
  Joanna Sheldon, Memo Spathis and Peter Watkins for their contribution to the questions and answers.
  Youth Section — Penny Earle and Kevin Brown.
  Children's Committee — Present Chairman, Peter Swift for his help on the section about babies and parents, Jennie Hirst, Barbara Elster and Susan Hordern.
  Parents' conference, Nene College, Northampton 1982.
Foreword — Dr Arnold Bloom and Sir Harry Secombe.
Line drawings — Julia Griffith-Jones.

  Illustrations and photographs with the assistance of Messrs Ames, Becton Dickinson, Eli Lilly, Genetics International, Hypoguard, MCP Pharmaceuticals, Mariner Medical, Sherwood Medical Industries, Medistron, Owen Mumford, Nordisk UK and Graseby Medical who all supply the needs of the diabetic.

  Contributors to questions; Clara Lowy for reading, amending and adding to pregnancy chapter; and Dr Matt Kiln for help with the Marathon question.

  Anonymous reviewers whose encouraging words made it worth continuing.

  Specialist nurses — Sally Bailey, Vivien Bowden, Maureen Brewin, Miranda Cowan and Pat McDowell.

Typing — Shirley Gunnell, Debbie Goodship and especially Lis Lawrence with a little help from Wang Wordprocessors.

Cathy Peck — whose idea it was and who managed to coax it into completion.

Long suffering patients who come to diabetic clinics at St Thomas' Hospital and Northampton General Hospital. Many of the questions have come from them and most of the solutions to problems have been worked out by the diabetics themselves. We are simply passing on their experience to others.

It is true to say that much of this book has been written by diabetics — for diabetics.

Introduction

What this book is not	**What this book is**
1 A medical textbook.	1 Questions of importance for anyone interested in diabetes.
2 A dictionary of diabetic terms.	2 Answers of clarity and simplicity.
3 A history of diabetes and its treatment.	3 Descriptions of biochemical changes.
4 A collection of case histories.	4 Facts about the problems diabetics face.
5 A battleplan for defeating diabetes.	5 Help in coming to terms with diabetes.
6 A list of miracle cures.	6 Descriptions of modern methods of making diabetes easier.
7 A formula for coping with a diabetic child.	7 Practical advice learnt from many parents of diabetic children.
8 Forecast of a cure for diabetes.	8 Surveys of current diabetes research and an informed guess about the future.

When diabetes suddenly hits you or a close relative, many unpleasant things come to mind ... injections, strict diets, urine tests, blindness. In fact most diabetics do not need injections, their diet is normal and wholesome, urine tests are going out of fashion and eye disease can now be successfully treated. However, a diabetic does have to learn to control his diabetes and he can only do this by understanding the condition. The diabetic gets much advice and help from nurses, doctors, dietitians and others, but it is his own decision how well he controls his condition. It is often said that the diabetic is his own doctor.

A lot of effort is being put into the education of diabetics and this book is part of that effort. There is a great deal of information to be learnt.

Diabetes is a complex disorder, and parts of this book reflect that complexity. Although some aspects of diabetes are hard to understand, most diabetics manage to lead full lives by incorporating their condition into normal work and activities. If you have just discovered that you or a close relative has diabetes, you will probably feel shocked and worried. This is not the time to try to learn about the more difficult aspects of the subject. But even at this early stage you (and your parents if you are a child) need to know certain basic facts. Once the initial shock-reaction is over and your own experience with diabetes increases, you will be ready to learn about the frills. Remember that *no one* involved in this subject (including doctors and nurses) ever stops learning more about it.

Throughout this book we have used the word diabetic to describe a person with diabetes. Some people feel that the word 'diabetic' should be used only as a description, as in 'diabetic clinic', and not as shorthand for a person with this condition. We do not ourselves feel the word diabetic is insulting in any way, and hope that our readers are not offended by it. It would be very cumbersome to write 'a person with diabetes' every time we meant 'diabetic'. Indeed, before making this decision we carried out a survey amongst the diabetic patients attending the clinic at St Thomas' Hospital; we found that the overwhelming majority were in favour of using this term, and no preferable alternative was suggested.

How to use this book

This book is a series of questions and answers, and it is not designed to be read from cover to cover. Some of the sections do stand on their own, in particular those describing the nature of diabetes, Chapter 1, Chapter 3 on diabetic control and Chapter 8 on long-term complications.

If you are a newly diagnosed diabetic, you may not be ready to come to grips with Chapter 9 on research but you may want to find out what is known about the causes of diabetes (p.11). If you have just started insulin injections you should read the following sections at an early stage:

Hypos (p.34).
Other illnesses (p.161).
Insulin (p.21).
Control and monitoring (p.95).
Blood glucose (p.97).
Driving (p.167).

More experienced diabetics will want to test us out in our answers in Chapter 4 on life with diabetes to see if our answers coincide with their experience. Parents of diabetic children will want to read Chapter 8 on the young diabetic.

There is bound to be some repetition in a book of this sort, but we think it is better to deal with similar topics under separate headings rather than ask the reader to shuttle from one end of the book to the other. We hope that at least we are consistent in our answers.

Feedback is one of the most important features of good diabetes care. This relies on the diabetic being honest with the doctor or nurse and vice versa. Not everyone will agree with the answers we give, but the book can only improve if you let us know when you disagree and have found our advice to be unhelpful. We would also like to know if there are important questions we have not dealt with. Please write to us c/o Harper & Row Ltd, 28 Tavistock Street, London WC2E 7PN, UK.

1

Diabetes

Introduction

This chapter opens with a description of how a diabetic might feel before his condition has been diagnosed and treated. Once treatment has been started the diabetic should feel perfectly well. We also make the point that older people may have diabetes and yet feel quite well in themselves. In this case the condition will be discovered only if they have a routine blood or urine test for sugar, and diabetes may therefore exist for many years without being discovered. Unfortunately, this 'mild', and undetected diabetes may, over a long period, lead to complications affecting eyes, nerves and blood vessels.

So there are two main types of diabetic:

a   younger people who feel unwell for a few weeks or months and may become very ill if they do not receive insulin;

b   older people who may have had diabetes for many years before it was discovered and who do not feel particularly unwell. In these people it is often discovered by chance and commonly responds well to diet or tablets — though sometimes insulin is needed.

There are other rare types of diabetes mentioned in this chapter.

We also answer very important questions about the central problem in diabetes, namely an increase in the amount of glucose (sugar) in the blood. We describe why this happens and why it may be dangerous.

Symptoms

1 Why does a young diabetic feel thirsty when the condition is first discovered?

The first signs of diabetes in a young person are thirst and loss of weight. These two symptoms are related and one leads to the other. The first thing to go wrong is the increased amount of urine. Normally we pass about $1\frac{1}{2}$ litres (just over 2 pints) of urine per day but a diabetic out of control may produce five times that amount. This continual loss of fluid dries out the body. The feeling of thirst is a warning that unless he drinks enough to replace the extra urine, he will soon be in trouble. Of course people who are not diabetic may also pass large amounts of urine. Every beer drinker knows the effect of 5 pints of best bitter. In this case the beer causes the extra urine whereas in diabetes the extra urine causes the thirst. The resulting thirst is usually mild in the early stages, and most people fail to realize its significance unless they happen to have a friend or relative with diabetes. An undiagnosed diabetic may take jugs of water up to bed and wake in the night to quench his thirst and pass water and still not realize that something is wrong. It would be a good thing if more people knew that unexplained thirst can be due to diabetes.

2 Why do diabetics often lose weight before their condition is brought under control?

One reason for the weight loss is simply the result of the large urine output, since this urine is loaded with sugar. An uncontrolled diabetic may lose in 24 hours as much as 1000 grams (approx 2 lb) of sugar. Anyone trying to lose weight knows that sugar = calories. These calories contained in the urine are lost to the body and are a drain on its resources —

hence the loss of weight. The 1000 grams of sugar lost are equivalent to 20 currant buns. Lack of insulin is another cause of weight loss in a diabetic who is out of control.

3   Why do some diabetics experience itching and soreness in the genital area?

A woman whose diabetes is out of control may be troubled by itching around the vagina. The technical name for this distressing symptom is pruritus vulvae. The equivalent complaint may be seen in men when the end of the penis becomes sore (balanitis). If the foreskin is also affected, it may become thickened (phimosis), which prevents the foreskin from being pulled back. This makes it impossible to keep the penis clean.

These problems are the result of infection with yeasts which thrive on the high concentration of sugar in this region. If the urine is kept free from sugar by good diabetic control, the itching and soreness will normally clear up. Anti-yeast cream from a doctor may speed up the improvement but this is only a holding measure while sugar is cleared from the urine.

4   Can the eyesight be affected early on in diabetes?

Most of the serious eye problems caused by diabetes are due to damage to the retina — retinopathy. (The retina is the 'photographic plate' at the back of the eye.)

Even minor changes in the retina take years to develop and are never seen early on in the disease in younger diabetics. Older people may have diabetes for years without being aware of it, and in those cases the retina may already be damaged by the time the condition is discovered.

The lens of the eye which is responsible for focussing the image on the retina can also be affected in diabetes. However, this is usually a temporary change and causes blurred vision which can be corrected by wearing glasses. The lens of the eye becomes swollen when diabetes is out of control and this makes the person short-sighted. As the diabetes comes under control, so the lens of the eye returns to its normal shape. A pair of glasses which was fitted for a swollen lens at a time of uncontrolled diabetes will no longer be suitable when the diabetes is brought under control. A new diabetic with blurred vision should wait a few months after things have settled down before visiting an optician for new spectacles. The blurred vision will probably improve on its own, and glasses may not be necessary.

In very rare cases the lens of the eye may be permanently damaged when diabetes is badly out of control (cataract).

5 Can diabetes be discovered by chance?

In young diabetics the diagnosis is usually made because the patient feels unwell and goes to the doctor.

In older people with no obvious medical problems, diabetes is often discovered as a result of a routine urine test — sometimes during an insurance examination. Once the diagnosis is made, the person may admit to feeling slightly thirsty or tired or to having itching (pruritus), but these symptoms are often not very dramatic, and may be put down to 'old age'. So in older people diabetes can take a milder form. Even though this form of diabetes seems to be a minor problem, it must still be taken very seriously. So-called 'mild' diabetes can still lead to problems with vision and circulation and in any case most people feel much better and more energetic once the diabetes is controlled. This can often be done by diet or diet and tablets though insulin injections are occasionally needed.

Types of diabetes

6 Are there different types of diabetes?

Yes. Diabetes exists in many different forms. Two main groups are recognized:

a Younger people (40 years or less) in whom the condition develops in a fairly dramatic way and when insulin injections are nearly always needed. About 30% of all diabetics fall into this category, known as Insulin Dependent Diabetics (or IDD for short).

b At the other end of the scale is the older person who develops diabetes with less obvious symptoms and who is often overweight. In this group insulin by injection is generally not needed and these patients are described as Non-Insulin Dependent Diabetics (or NIDD).

There are plenty of exceptions to this rule. Occasionally, young diabetics can be well controlled with diet or tablets and quite a large number of people who develop diabetes late in life are much better off on insulin injections.

7 *What is diabetes insipidus?*

The only connection between diabetes insipidus and the usual form of diabetes (mellitus) is that people with both conditions pass large amounts of urine. Diabetes insipidus is a rare condition due to an abnormality in the pituitary gland and not the pancreas. One disorder does not lead to the other.

8 *I have recently been given steroid treatment (prednisone) for severe arthritis. My joints are better but my doctor has now found sugar in my urine and tells me I am diabetic. Is this likely to be permanent?*

Steroids are very effective treatment for a number of conditions but they may cause side-effects — as you have just discovered. One of these side-effects is to cause diabetes which can usually be controlled with tablets (e.g. glibenclamide) and insulin is not usually required. When you stop steroid therapy there is a good chance that the diabetes will go away completely. However, you *may* have been a mild diabetic without knowing it before you started steroids in which case you will need to continue some form of diabetic treatment indefinitely.

9 *I am told that other hormones apart from insulin may cause diabetes. Please could you enlarge on this?*

It is a deficiency of the hormone insulin that leads to diabetes. If certain other hormones (chemical messengers) are produced in excessive amounts then diabetes may result.

Thus people who produce too much thyroid hormone (thyrotoxicosis) may develop mild diabetes which clears up when the thyroid is restored to normal. Also, thyrotoxicosis and diabetes tend to run together in families, and people with one condition are more likely to develop the other.

Sometimes a person will produce excessive quantities of steroid hormones (Cushing's disease), and this may lead to diabetes (see previous question). Acromegaly is a condition where excess quantities of growth hormone are produced and this often leads to mild diabetes.

10 Can a severe illness cause diabetes?

Any serious condition (e.g. coronary thrombosis or severe injuries from a traffic accident) may lead to diabetes. This is because most of the hormones produced in response to stress tend to have the opposite effect to insulin and cause the glucose level in the blood to rise. Most people simply produce more insulin to keep the blood glucose stable. However, in some cases if the reserves of insulin are inadequate the blood glucose level will climb. Such a person is a temporary diabetic, and the glucose level will usually return to normal once the stress is over. However, they will have an increased risk of becoming a permanent diabetic later on in life.

11 My wife has just given birth to a baby boy who weighed 4.3 kg (9½ lb) at birth. Apparently she may have been a diabetic while she was pregnant. Is this likely to happen again with her next baby?

Women who give birth to heavy babies (over 4 kg, or 9 lb) may have had a raised blood glucose level during pregnancy. This extra glucose crosses into the unborn baby, who responds by producing extra insulin of its own. The combination of excess glucose and excess insulin makes the unborn baby grow fat and bloated. Once it has been born and cut off from its supply of glucose from the mother, the baby may then become hypoglycaemic (develop a low glucose concentration in the blood). These fat babies of diabetic mothers (even mild diabetics) are definitely at risk.

Mothers who become diabetic during pregnancy and who then return to normal after their babies are born are called *gestational diabetics*. Once the problem has been identified the mother will have to keep a close check on her blood glucose during any subsequent pregnancy. Provided it is kept strictly normal (usually insulin is needed for this), the baby will be a normal weight and will not be at risk.

Women who are diabetic during pregnancy are more likely to become diabetic later in life.

12 *I have had to go to hospital for repeated attacks of pancreatitis and now have diabetes. I am told these two conditions are related*

Pancreatitis means that the pancreas has become inflamed and this can be a very painful and unpleasant illness. The pancreas is the gland which among other things produces insulin and if it becomes badly inflamed and scarred it may not be able to produce enough of this hormone. Sometimes during or after an attack of pancreatitis a patient may become diabetic and need tablets or insulin to keep the blood glucose controlled. This form of diabetes is usually but not always permanent.

Causes of diabetes

13 *Why have I got diabetes?*

The short answer is that your pancreas is no longer making enough insulin for your body's needs. The long answer as to why this has happened to *you* is not so well understood. However, there are a few clues. Diabetes may run in families (p.14). Other possible causes are discussed in this section. It is not a rare condition. In England about 1 in 50 people have diabetes and the chances increase with age. About 2 in 1000 children under 16 years of age are diabetic.

14 *Is diabetes caused by a virus?*

Despite a vast amount of research throughout the world the cause of diabetes is not known (p.256). It is known that in some families there is a tendency towards diabetes (p.14) and that the disease in young people often develops when triggered off by some infection or cold. Some people suspect that a certain virus could actually cause diabetes but there is no proof. If a virus is the cause, it is probably a common one (like Cocksackie B) which leads to diabetes only in susceptible people (i.e. those who have inherited some diabetic tendency). There is no 'diabetes virus' and you cannot catch diabetes like chicken pox. Research workers have suggested that full-blown diabetes may not be discovered for several years after the infection has occurred. Diabetes in older people is probably nothing to do with a virus infection.

15 Can fatness cause diabetes?

If the tendency towards diabetes is present, then fatness (obesity) may bring on the disease. This does not happen in young people, but is a common cause of diabetes in middle-aged or older people (p.71). In most cases this type of diabetes can be controlled by dieting and weight loss. Many fat people with diabetes find it hard to stick to a diet; others find that strict dieting alone is insufficient to lower the blood glucose and have to take tablets or insulin injections. This is second-best as the sensible and safe treatment for an obese older diabetic is *weight loss*.

16 Can a bad shock bring on diabetes?

Sometimes diabetes develops soon after a major disturbance in life, such as a bereavement, a heart attack, or a bad accident and the diabetes is blamed on the upset. This is not really the case, as insulin failure in the pancreas takes a long time to develop. However, a bad shock may stress the system and bring on diabetes a bit earlier if the insulin supply is already running low.

17 Do large babies cause their mother to be diabetic?

No. It's the other way round. In pregnancy even very mild diabetes, which may not be detected without special tests, may result in an overweight baby. In any woman who has given birth to a baby weighing more than 4 kg (9 lb), the possibility of diabetes should be considered by her doctors. If a mother is diabetic during pregnancy but recovers soon after her baby is born, she does carry a slightly increased risk of diabetes for the rest of her life. The baby itself does not carry this risk. (More details are given on p.198.)

18   Can diabetes be prevented?

No. At the present time, if you are going to get diabetes, you get diabetes. It is possible, under certain circumstances, to identify some people who are not diabetic but who have a very high risk of becoming so within a year of so. Various drugs have been tried to prevent diabetes in these high-risk people, but so far with no success.

19   Can tablets or medicines cause diabetes or make diabetes worse?

Yes; there are several drugs in common usage that either cause diabetes as an unwanted side-effect or make existing diabetes worse. The most important group of such medicines are hormones. Hormones are substances produced by special glands in the body and insulin from the pancreas is itself a hormone. Some hormones have an anti-insulin effect and one of these, a steroid hormone, is sometimes used in treating medical conditions, such as severe asthma or rheumatoid arthritis. The most commonly used steroid is prednisolone which opposes insulin and therefore tends to cause the level of sugar in the blood to rise. Steroids in large doses will often cause diabetes which usually gets better when the steroids are stopped (p.9). The contraceptive pill is another type of steroid hormone with a very mild anti-insulin effect. Sometimes diabetics on insulin find they have to give themselves more insulin if they are on the pill. Glucagon is a hormone from the pancreas with a very strong anti-insulin effect. It is used to correct a severe insulin reaction (p.37). Apart from other hormones, certain medicines may have an anti-insulin effect. In particular diuretics (water tablets) which make people pass extra amounts of urine often cause a mild form of diabetes. Cough syrups made up of a concentrated sugar solution are not recommended in diabetes, but in practice they do not seem to cause any harm unless taken in excess.

Inheritance

20   Does diabetes run in families?

Diabetes is a common disorder affecting about 1 out of 50 people. So, in any large family more than one person may be affected, simply by chance alone. However, certain families do seem to carry a very strong tendency for diabetes. The worst example of this is a whole tribe of American Indians (the Pima) where over half its members develop diabetes by the time they reach middle age. Genes are the parts of a human cell that decide which characteristics you inherit from your parents. The particular genes that you get from each parent are a matter of chance — in other words whether you grow up with your father's big feet or your mother's blue eyes. Similarly it is a matter of chance whether you pass on the genes carrying the tendency for diabetes to one of your children. It is only the tendency to diabetes which you *may* pass on and the full-blown condition will not develop unless something else causes the insulin cells in the pancreas to fail. If you are a diabetic parent there is probably a 1 in 100 chance that your child will be diabetic by the age of 30. This is a small but increased risk compared with normal.

21   I am 16 and have been diabetic for 5 years. Why has my identical twin brother not got diabetes?

A large study has been carried out at King's College Hospital, London, where they have been collecting examples of identical twins for over 10 years. Their results show an interesting difference between young diabetics who need insulin and older diabetics who usually manage on diet or tablets. If you have an identical twin who is a young diabetic on insulin, then you only have a 50% chance of becoming diabetic yourself. On the other hand, the identical twin of a middle-aged diabetic who does not need insulin is almost 100% certain to get the same sort of diabetes. So in your case your twin brother has an evens chance of becoming diabetic.

Incidentally, the doctors at the Diabetic Department at King's College Hospital are keen to hear about any cases of diabetes in identical twins. If you are not already on their books why not ask your doctor to tell them about your case?

Physiology

22 What is the pancreas?

The pancreas is a gland situated in the upper part of the abdomen connected by a fine tube to the intestine. It releases digestive juices which are mixed with the food soon after it leaves the stomach. They are needed for food to be digested and absorbed into the body. This part of the pancreas has nothing to do with diabetes.

The pancreas also produces a number of hormones which are released directly into the bloodstream — unlike digestive juices which pass into the intestine. The most important of these hormones is insulin, lack of which causes diabetes. The other important hormone produced by the pancreas is glucagon which has the opposite action to insulin and may be used in correcting serious hypos (p.37).

23 Is diabetes a disease of modern times?

No. The earliest detailed description of diabetes was made 2000 years ago. Diabetes appears to be more common than in the past. This is partly because mild cases which would not have been picked up are nowadays detected by routine check-ups. There is a suggestion that diabetes in younger people may be occurring more frequently, but as yet there is no definite proof for this theory.

24 Why does the body need insulin?

Without insulin the body cannot make full use of food that is eaten. Normally, food is eaten, taken into the body and broken down into simple units which then provide fuel for all the activities of the body. These simple units also provide building blocks for growth or replacing worn-out parts. In diabetes food is broken down as normal, but because of shortage of insulin the fuel and building blocks cannot be used properly. Insulin is sometimes likened to the funnel for getting petrol into the fuel tank of a car or to a key which opens the door and allows food to reach where it is needed.

25 How does insulin control the supply of fuel?

Food is a mixture of complex materials which are absorbed into the body and broken down to various simple chemicals. This takes place in the liver which can be regarded as a food-processing factory. Glucose is one of the simple chemicals made in the liver from all carbohydrate foods. In the absence of insulin, glucose pours out of the liver into the bloodstream. Insulin switches off this outpouring of glucose from the liver and causes glucose to be stored in the liver as starch or glycogen.

Insulin also helps glucose to get inside the cells where it is used as a fuel. So if there is not enough insulin, glucose will pour out of the liver into the bloodstream and have difficulty getting into the cells. This causes a build-up of glucose in the blood. Insulin has a similar effect on amino acids and fatty acids which are the breakdown products of protein and fat, respectively.

26 How do people who are not diabetic get their insulin?

Insulin is stored in the pancreas and immediately the blood glucose level starts to rise after eating, insulin is released into the bloodstream. It is taken straight to the liver where it has the important effect of stopping glucose production and favouring its storage. The level of glucose in the blood then falls and as it does so, insulin production is switched off. So people who are not diabetic have a very sensitive system for keeping the amount of glucose in the blood at a steady level.

The slightest rise in blood glucose causes insulin to be produced. This in turn brings down the glucose level, and the insulin is switched off.

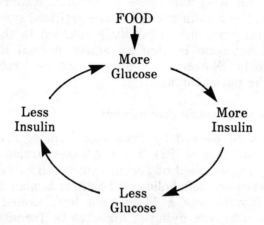

FOOD
More Glucose
More Insulin
Less Glucose
Less Insulin

In diabetics this system is faulty. Mild diabetics have some insulin but the pancreas cannot produce it fast enough, or in sufficient amounts, so the blood glucose level goes up. More severe diabetics have little or no insulin of their own and injections of insulin are needed to try to keep the blood glucose level normal.

Obviously, an injection of insulin once or twice a day is not as efficient at regulating blood glucose as the pancreas which can switch insulin supply on or off at a moment's notice in response to minute fluctuations.

27 *Can a diabetic on insulin keep his blood glucose at a normal level?*

Yes, although it may not be easy and can only be done by means of a balancing act. There are three main things which affect the blood glucose: (i) food (which puts it up); (ii) insulin; and (iii) exercise (which both bring it down). Any form of stress, in particular an illness like flu, puts up the blood glucose. The only way of learning how to balance the blood glucose level is by trial and error. This means making a lot of measurements and discovering how various foods and forms of exercise alter the blood glucose.

In the past diabetics were brought into hospital to be 'stabilized' on a certain dose of insulin. Experience has shown that the insulin needed in the artificial surroundings of a hospital ward may bear little relation to the amount needed in someone leading an active normal life in the outside world. Nowadays, diabetes can be 'stabilized' at home by the patient himself.

28   When was insulin discovered?

Insulin was discovered by Frederick Banting and Charles Best in the summer of 1921. The work was carried out in the Physiology Department of Toronto University while most of the staff were on their holidays. The first human diabetic to be given insulin was a 14-year-old boy, named Leonard Thompson, who was dying of diabetes in Toronto General Hospital. This was an historic event, representing the beginning of modern diabetic treatment. It was then up to the chemists to transform the production of insulin into an industrial process on a vast scale.

Related conditions

29   Do other diseases increase the chances of getting diabetes?

Yes. These can be grouped as follows:

1   Glandular disorders:
    Thyrotoxicosis (overactive thyroid)
    Acromegaly (excess growth hormone)
    Cushing's disease (excess steroid hormone).
2   Disease of the pancreas:
    Pancreatitis
    Cancer of the pancreas

Surgical removal of the pancreas (for one or other of
above)
Haemochromatosis (iron overload)
Cystic fibrosis (a childhood disorder).
3   Virus disease:
German measles ⎞
Mumps   ⎬ rarely lead to diabetes.
Cocksackie   ⎠
4   Stress:
Heart attack
Pneumonia
Major surgical operation.
The diabetes usually clears up when the stress is removed.

2

Treatment

Introduction

Here we describe different ways of controlling diabetes. In younger patients there is usually no choice and they need to start insulin injections fairly soon but in older people found to be diabetic the eventual form of treatment they will need may not be obvious at the outset. Provided they are not feeling terribly ill this sort of patient is usually put on a diet and this alone will have a dramatic effect on their condition, especially in obese patients who manage to get their weight down. If diet on its own fails to control diabetes, tablets are usually tried next. These may be very effective but tablets do not always work and in such cases insulin is the only alternative. With the new syringes now available, insulin injections have become much less of a burden.

We have a section on insulin pumps. These devices are effective but demand a great deal of co-operation from the patient and a 24-hour back-up from the hospital. For this reason insulin pumps are only used in specialized research centres. However, there will be great advances in the technology of insulin pumps and it is likely that over the next few years they will be more widely available.

The next section is one of the most important parts of this book. This concerns the problem of hypos — in other words, a *low* blood sugar. They usually affect diabetics on insulin, but can happen to those taking tablets. It is the fear of hypos that prevents some diabetics from controlling their blood sugar carefully. Doctors are often criticized for not giving new diabetics enough information on hypos. So, if you have just started insulin treatment, *read this section* (p.34).

We have included a number of questions on diet, dealing firstly with general principles on eating, which apply to all diabetics. We then answer a number of questions about food and eating patterns of particular importance to diabetics on insulin. We do not aim to go into diet in exhaustive detail and if you want more information we recommend the following books:

> *The Diabetics' Diet Book* by Dr Jim Mann, published by Martin Dunitz.
> *Carbohydrate Countdown* (BDA Publications).
> *Better Cookery for Diabetics* by Jill Metcalfe (BDA Publications).
> *Cooking the New Diabetic Way* (BDA Publications).
> *The Vegetarian on a Diet* by Margaret Cousins and Jill Metcalfe, published by Thorson's Publishers.
> *The Diabetic's Cookbook* by Roberta Longstaff SRD and Dr Jim Mann, published by Martin Dunitz.

Most people with diabetes and especially parents of diabetic children long for a miracle cure and this explains why we have been sent so many questions about unorthodox methods of treatment. We have tried to answer these questions in a sensitive manner but there is no escaping the fact that for a diabetic child, insulin is the only miracle cure and that is how it was regarded when discovered in 1921.

Insulin

1   Where does insulin come from?

Insulin is obtained from the most easily available large animals, i.e. cow and pig. Insulin from these animals differs only slightly from human insulin and to the vast majority of diabetics these differences are not important. Insulin identical with the human variety has now been made, either by modifying pork insulin or by persuading a bacterium to make it by means of genetic engineering. There is still no evidence that this human insulin is better for the average diabetic than the highly purified beef or pork insulins. However, some people may prefer the idea of having insulin from their own species.

2 How is the long-acting insulin made?

The first insulin to be made was ordinary soluble insulin. Injected under the skin, this lasts for about 6 hours and is called short-acting insulin. Various modifications were made to this original insulin so that it would be absorbed more slowly from an injection under the skin. By incorporating protamine or zinc into the insulin a single injection could be made to last from 12 up to 36 hours. For many years a single, daily injection was advised by many doctors but it was then found that this is not a good way to control the variations in blood glucose that occur during the day. Nowadays most diabetics who need insulin take a mixture of short and long-acting insulins twice a day.

3 Is there any real advantage in using the newer, more purified insulins?

Most patients do not get any obvious benefit if they change from the older insulins to new, pure varieties. Some people develop unsightly hollows if they repeatedly inject the older types of insulin into the same site. Highly purified insulins often do the opposite and cause lumps to form if the site of the injection is never changed. Once the lumps develop, people tend to go on injecting into them as it is convenient and painless. However, this is not a good idea as insulin is absorbed slowly and unpredictably from these fatty lumps — and they have an unpleasant appearance. The lumps can be avoided by carefully injecting into a different place each time.

4 *My doctor is considering changing me from one to two insulin injections per day. Will the second interfere with my social life — eating out, etc.?*

No. The second injection should make life more flexible. Most people on one injection a day find they need a meal in the late afternoon, around 6 to 7 p.m. With a second injection, this meal can be delayed for several hours with the insulin given shortly beforehand. With the new plastic syringes it is easy to give oneself insulin even when eating out.

5 *Sometimes after I inject my insulin I get a rash and itchiness all over my body. My doctor says that I am allergic to the insulin and has changed my insulin from Lente to Monotard. Is this form of allergy common?*

The older, less pure insulins (such as Lente) sometimes cause an itchy rash at the site of the injection. This hardly ever happens with the newer, highly purified insulins (such as Monotard) which do not stimulate the body to produce many antibodies. Very occasionally diabetics may develop an allergy to one of the additives to insulin such as protamine or zinc.

6 *I have been taking insulin for 20 years. Recently, I noticed red lumps after injecting into my legs. These lumps do not appear anywhere else. Have you any idea what they can be?*

In the past when insulin was not as highly purified as it is nowadays, it was quite common for red, itchy lumps to appear at the site of injections. This was probably due to impurities in the insulin and is not often seen nowadays. Another cause of painful lumps at the injection site is that the needle is not going in deeply enough so that the insulin is being forced *in between* the layers of skin rather than into the fat below. This may happen when people change to new plastic syringes with very short needles. These really have to be injected straight down at right angles to the skin rather than at an oblique angle. However, after 20 years on insulin, neither of these explanations seems very likely so there is no simple answer to your question.

7 Is it possible for a diabetic to take his insulin injection immediately after a meal rather than before?

People who are not diabetic start to produce insulin at the very beginning of a meal. Since it takes some time for insulin (injected) to be absorbed, it is usual to have an insulin injection before a meal. This is the best way of keeping the blood glucose balanced.

8 How long before eating should I have my insulin injection?

With the older, less purified insulin, diabetics were often advised to have their insulin more than half-an-hour before eating. However, highly purified insulins tend to be absorbed more rapidly, and if the delay between insulin and food is too long you run the risk of a hypo (p.34). Now that most diabetics are measuring their own blood glucose they are able to keep this level closer to normal, so there is less leeway before the blood glucose falls too low. Therefore it is sensible to inject your insulin and start eating within 15 or 20 minutes.

9 When I was first diagnosed I was put on insulin but now the dosage has been decreased. The doctor tells me I am in the 'honeymoon period' of diabetes. What does this mean?

Most people need a reduction in their insulin dose soon after the diagnosis is made. This is due to partial recovery of the insulin-producing cells of the pancreas. During this period hypos are often a problem but on the whole it is easy to control the blood glucose during the 'honeymoon'. The 'honeymoon period' usually comes to a sudden end within a few months, often during a bad cold or some other stress to the insulin-producing cells. However, the 'honeymoon period' is a good thing and improves the chances of successful long-term diabetic control.

10   *When I developed diabetes I was started on insulin but*
     kept having hypos and 3 months ago I came off insulin.
     Why was I given it in the first place?

Presumably you were given insulin because your doctors
thought you needed it. Most diabetics under 40 years old
who have ketones in their urine are likely to need insulin and
tend to be started on this without any delay. After having
insulin for a week or so, it is quite common for the diabetic to
be troubled by hypos, in which case the insulin has to be
reduced. Sometimes even tiny doses of insulin cause hypos
during this 'honeymoon period' (see previous question) and
the injections have to be stopped completely. The
'honeymoon period' may occasionally last as long as 6
months.

11   *How far have scientists got in producing human insulin*
     from bacteria?

Eli Lilly, who were the first firm to manufacture insulin on a
large scale in 1927, have now persuaded bacteria to produce
insulin that is exactly the same as human insulin. This new
'human' insulin was launched in UK in September 1982 but
there is still no evidence that it acts differently from other
purified insulins.
    Novo were the first company to make highly purified pork
insulin and they have managed to modify this so that it is
identical with human insulin. So if you want humanized
insulin you have the choice of getting it either from pigs or
bacteria. Insulin made from bacteria does *not* give rise to
infection!

12   *I am on two injections a day. Sometimes I find it*
     inconvenient to take my evening injection. Can I skip it
     and have a meal containing no carbohydrate?

No, you cannot skip the evening injection. When the effect of
your morning injection wears out your blood glucose level
will rise even if you have no carbohydrate to eat. Nowadays
by using a plastic syringe, injections are much less
inconvenient. If you are eating out, you can give your injection just before your meal.

13   What should I do if I suddenly realize I have missed an injection?

It is quite easy to forget to give your injection or even worse to be unable to remember whether you have had your injection. If this happens you should measure your blood sugar to help you decide what to do next. If the blood sugar is high (more than 10 mmol/l) you probably did forget your injection and you should have some insulin as soon as possible. The dose depends on how close you are to the *next* injection time. If your blood glucose is normal or low (7 or less) you probably did have your injection even if you have forgotten doing it. It would be safest to check your blood again before the next meal and if it is high have an extra dose of short-acting insulin. If you are using urine tests as a guide then the urine test will probably show 2% glucose if the injection has been missed.

14   Does the timing of injections matter? Can a diabetic who is on two injections a day take them at 10.00 a.m. and 4.00 p.m.?

It is best to have insulin shortly before a meal (p.24) and if you have your main meals in the middle of the morning and in the afternoon then you could try giving insulin at those times. You may find that an afternoon injection may not last the 18 hours until the next morning and that is why most diabetics try to keep their two injections approximately 12 hours apart.

15   I am interested in getting a small cooler box with a frozen block. Would this be suitable for carrying insulin abroad?

Fortunately insulin is very stable. It is usually recommended that it should be stored in a cool place and it will 'go off' if left in hot sunlight or in tropical conditions. However, during a 2–3 week holiday abroad it is perfectly all right to keep insulin bottles in ordinary luggage or handbags without any special measures for cooling.

16 I have unsightly lumps and hollows on my upper thighs where I inject my insulin. Could I have plastic surgery to make my thighs smooth again?

One of the main practical differences between older insulins and the new highly purified type is the effect they have if injected daily into the same site. Highly purified insulins tend to cause fatty lumps, while the older types lead to hollows as well as lumps. Both are unsightly and they can cause problems in diabetic control because they alter the rate at which insulin is absorbed. They are best avoided by moving the injection site each time — up and down each thigh and across the abdomen. If you have lumps already they will go away in due course if you stop injecting into them. The hollows (usually due to older insulin) can be filled out by changing to highly purified insulins and injecting these around the outside of the hollows until they gradually fill out. Plastic surgery is not recommended.

17 Should I increase my insulin over Christmas to cope with the extra food I shall be eating?

At Christmas everyone (including diabetics) eats more and it is best to accept this. Extra food does need extra insulin and it is up to you to try to discover how much to increase your dose. The extra insulin is best taken in quick-acting form shortly before the meal.

Don't forget the effect of exercise on the blood sugar — the traditional afternoon stroll following Christmas dinner is probably a good idea.

18 I have been a diabetic for 9 months and attend the diabetic clinic every month to have my insulin dose adjusted. How long does it usually take before doctors get you balanced?

This is an interesting question, as it assumes that it is up to the *doctors* to balance *your* diabetes. Of course the doctors and nurses in the clinic must provide you with all the help and information you need but in the end it is *your* diabetes for *you* to control. Good diabetic control depends not just on the dose of insulin but the site of the injection, the timing and type of food and the amount of exercise. These are things that the doctor himself has no direct control over. Most diabetics are beginning to get their blood glucose under control in a week or two.

19 *As I am mixing neutral and isophane insulin 50/50 I wonder whether I should change to Initard?*

There are three brands of insulin containing fixed proportions of short- and medium-acting insulin: Mixtard (neutral 30%, isophane 70%) and Initard (50% of each) and Rapitard (25% neutral, 75% crystalline). If you changed to Initard you would gain by making the drawing up of the insulin more convenient but you would lose the flexibility and the ability to adjust the proportions if necessary. People who use Mixtard, Initard or Rapitard should keep a bottle of pure quick-acting insulin for use in illness or in case a quick boost is needed.

20 *Is my insulin requirement likely to vary at different times of the year because of the weather?*

Several diabetics have remarked that their dose of insulin needs to be altered in very hot weather — some need to give themselves more insulin and others less. This is probably because people react in different ways to a heatwave. There is a tendency to eat less and take less exercise in tropical conditions. However, because blood flow to the skin is increased in warm temperatures this could speed up the absorption of the injected insulin and mean that a given dose will not last as long. Everyone is different and you will have to find out for yourself how hot weather affects your own blood glucose.

21 *I have recently changed from soluble insulin to Actrapid and Insulatard and since then I have been having headaches, face flushes and nausea. These clear up if I decrease my dose of insulin but then I show a*

quarter percent sugar in my urine. Have you any idea what can be causing these symptoms?

If this was an allergy to the new insulin you would react in the same way to a small dose as you would to a large dose and in any case your new insulins are highly purified and unlikely to cause an allergic response. Since you are feeling better on a reduced dose of insulin, the unpleasant feelings you describe are probably due to a low blood sugar. The urine test at a quarter per cent could well be misleading and you could easily sort things out by measuring your own blood glucose at the time when you feel unwell. You probably do need to have less of the new insulin.

22 *Is it all right for me, as a diabetic on insulin, to have a lie-in on Sunday or must I get up and have my injection and breakfast at the normal time?*

Like many of the answers in this book, the best advice is try it and see. Try missing out your morning injection and breakfast and measure your blood glucose when you get up 3 or 4 hours late. If it is well below 10 mmol/l, all well and good, but if the blood glucose is higher than 10 mmol/l it means that you should not have missed your insulin. Alternatively try to get someone else to give you your morning injection and bring you up some breakfast.

23 *When one's insulin requirements decrease over the years, does this mean that the pancreas has gradually started to produce more natural insulin than when one was younger?*

No. It is most unlikely that after many years of diabetes the pancreas will start to produce natural insulin. However, this reduction in dose in older people is well recognized. It could be that you were having more insulin than you really needed in the past. Since the introduction of blood glucose measurement many people are found to be having too much insulin — or sometimes too much at one time of the day and not enough at another. Other possible explanations for older people needing less insulin are that they eat less food or because of hormonal changes.

24 *While I take every precaution to ensure that I never miss an injection I am convinced that one day, as a result of carelessness or an accident, this may happen. Can you tell me what I should do if I miss an injection?*

Be assured that many diabetics (even the most organized) forget to have their injection once in a while and come to no harm. If you realize that you have missed an injection, provided that you feel all right, no serious problem will arise. Give yourself a dose of short-acting insulin before the next meal.

In case of accident (especially if you are unconscious) then it is of course vital that the people looking after you know you are a diabetic. For this reason you should always wear an information bracelet or necklace (e.g. SOS or Medicalert). Sadly, many diabetics fail to take this simple precaution which could be life saving.

25 *I have two injections a day: morning and evening. I keep regular times for breakfast and evening tea but I would like to vary the time I take lunch. What effect would this have on my diabetic control?*

This is a difficult problem for a diabetic on insulin. Because of the morning injection, people often tend to feel hypo if they are late for lunch. If the morning injection is mainly intermediate-acting insulin (e.g. Monotard or Insulatard), you may be able to delay your lunch a little provided you have a mid-morning snack.

26 *Sometimes I suffer from a poor appetite. Is it all right for me to reduce my insulin dose on such occasions?*

Yes, that is perfectly acceptable provided that you don't miss out completely on a main meal. You will have to find out for yourself (by measuring blood glucose) how much you should reduce the insulin for a particular amount of food. If you are underweight do not reduce your food intake too drastically. On the other hand, overweight diabetics need to reduce both food intake and insulin.

The pump

27   *I hear a lot about insulin pumps for treating diabetics.
      Doctors in my own clinic never seem very keen on the
      idea. How do pumps work and are they a good form of
      treatment?*

First, an explanation of why insulin pumps have been
developed. People who are not diabetic release a very small
amount of insulin into the bloodstream throughout the day
and then every time they eat any food the pancreas produces
extra insulin. In this way the blood glucose is kept at a very
steady level. Without the constant 'background' insulin in
between meals, the blood glucose levels would slowly rise. It
is not easy to get the same pattern of background insulin
plus extra squirts for meals in a diabetic who has to inject
insulin under the skin. Insulin pumps are an attempt to copy
this normal pattern. They consist of a slow-running motor
attached to a syringe filled with a solution of insulin. The
insulin is pumped down a fine-bore tube into a needle which
is inserted under the skin and strapped in place. The pump
also has a device for giving additional boosts of insulin before
meals.

A few centres in the USA have developed very elaborate
pumps which can be programmed to deliver insulin boosts at
planned times of day.

Many hundreds of diabetics have successfully controlled
their blood glucose with an insulin pump. However, the
complaint is always made that they are cumbersome
machines which have to be carried about all day long. Insulin
pumps (*see* Plate 1) are also complicated to manage and most
centres which give them to diabetics need a full-time nurse
simply to instruct the patient and give instant advice when
things go wrong. Diabetics sometimes get the impression
that if only they were given an insulin pump all their
problems would be solved and their diabetes would look
after itself. In practice, however, patients using pumps have
to do more blood glucose measurements and need to make
regular adjustments to their dose of insulin. Like all
machines insulin pumps are capable of going wrong and

unless you have a close link with a specialist centre, you are better off with a plastic syringe and a bottle of insulin.

However, a lot of work is being done to try to make insulin pumps smaller, simpler and more reliable. The day may come when diabetics needing insulin will be issued with the pump as a routine. That day is still a few years off.

28 My diabetes is well controlled. Should I be thinking of buying a pump?

Probably not, if your diabetes really is well controlled. The pump is presently only used in a small number of diabetic clinics throughout the UK. Insulin pumps can only be used in conjunction with an expert team who can provide 24-hour cover in case of emergencies. Without such technical back-up, it is not really feasible to embark on pump therapy.

Research has shown that, if you are the sort of person who achieves good control by giving insulin with a standard insulin syringe, then you would probably be able to do *slightly* better by using a pump. However, if your control is normally erratic then fixing you up with a pump is not likely to improve matters.

29 How much do pumps cost?

Pumps are expensive. The cheapest in common use is the Mill Hill Infuser which costs around £300. There are additional running costs:

Infusion cannula (line and needle attached) £128 pa.
Battery £125 pa.
Saline £22 pa.

This comes to a total of £275 pa with insulin and syringes on top of that. New, more compact pumps will probably cost twice as much as the Mill Hill model. Some insulin pumps incorporate a memory and can be programmed to give a different dose of insulin at different times of the day. These are likely to cost more than £1000.

30   Do pumps mean less injections?

One advantage of giving insulin by a pump is that you can insert the cannula (fine tube plus needle) and leave it in place for about 3 days on end. However, it is not easy to have a shower or bath while strapped to a pump. Nor are many forms of sport compatible with wearing a pump. So, in practice, the needle will have to be replaced on most days.

31   What are the main difficulties of using a pump for giving insulin?

The main problem with pumps is that, like all machines, they are capable of going wrong. One reason for the high cost of insulin pumps is the need to build into the design a warning system to alert the user to a mechanical fault. If the pump suddenly stops, the user will rapidly go into a state of complete insulin lack and may quickly develop ketoacidosis.

Since the needle remains under the skin it acts as a foreign body and may set up a focus of infection leading to an abscess. The cannula must only be inserted after careful cleaning of the skin.

From the user's point of view, the main disadvantage of the pump is the fact that it has to be worn day and night. This is obviously more inconvenient than the ordinary injections which are over and done with. Many people dislike the pump which they find a constant reminder of their diabetes.

32   I have heard a news report about a nurse from the North of England who has been fitted with an implantable insulin pump. Could you please give me more details?

The woman in question is an extremely unstable diabetic. The pump (called an Infusaide) works by draining insulin out of a reservoir down a fine tube into a blood vessel at a constant rate. The reservoir is filled by an injection into the skin every 2 weeks or so. At present these pumps are not available for general use and can only be considered in those cases where a person's life is being completely disrupted by unstable diabetes. Infection may cause serious problems and there may be other difficulties yet to be discovered. The Infusaide pumps are very expensive — £4000 or more.

Hypos

33 Since my wife has been started on insulin she has had 'funny turns'. What is the cause of this?

Your wife's funny turns are due to a low blood glucose. The medical name for this is hypoglycaemia and most people call it HYPO for short. The feelings people have when they are hypo are due to two things: (i) the brain itself cannot work properly if the blood glucose falls below a certain level — usually 2 mmol/l; and (ii) the body reacts to a low blood sugar by producing hormones (mainly adrenaline) which increase the blood glucose. When the brain is affected by a low blood glucose level, it may cause weakness of the legs, double or blurred vision, confusion, headache and in severe cases loss of consciousness and convulsions. The adrenaline causes sweating, rapid heartbeat and feelings of panic and anxiety. Children often describe a 'dizzy feeling in the tummy' or just 'tiredness' when they are hypo. Most diabetics find it hard to describe exactly how they feel when hypo but the proof is that the blood glucose is low (less than 2.5 mmol/l) and the feeling is quickly put right by taking some form of glucose or sugar.

34 I am taking soluble and isophane insulin twice a day and am getting hypos 2–3 hours after my evening meal. As I live alone this has been worrying me. What can I do?

Anyone who is having frequent hypos at a particular time of day can easily put this right by adjusting their insulin. In this case you are having hypos at the time when the evening dose of soluble insulin is working. You should reduce the amount of soluble insulin you take in the evening until you stop having hypos at that time. Hypos *before* the evening meal could be corrected by reducing the dose of morning intermediate-acting (isophane) insulin.

35 My daughter is diabetic and sometimes turns very nasty and short tempered. Is this due to the insulin?

Yes, probably — though it is not the only cause of bad moods in teenage girls! The only way to find out is try to persuade her to have a blood glucose measurement during her bad moods. If it is low (3 mmol/l or less) then some glucose should restore her good nature. Because the brain is affected by a low blood glucose level, irrational behaviour is common during a hypo. Your daughter may forcibly deny that she is hypo and resist taking the glucose her body needs. If you are firm and do not panic you will be able to talk her into taking the glucose (Lucozade can be useful here) and she will soon be back to normal).
NB: Children can also become irritable if their blood glucose is very high.

36 My 8-year-old son often complains of feeling tired after recovering from a hypo. Is this usual and what is the best way to overcome it?

There are many different warnings of an oncoming hypo. These include shaking, sweating, pins and needles around the lips and tongue, palpitation, a sense of hunger, headache, double vision, slow thinking and, in some children, vomiting. To this list may be added a sense of tiredness and heaviness, and some people yawn repeatedly when hypo. There are other feelings which individuals recognize for themselves — often the parent or spouse of a diabetic can tell by a certain characteristic expression or gesture.

Apart from headache, these feelings usually vanish within five minutes of taking glucose. It is unusual to feel tired for a long time after a hypo but if your son does so, you should first check his blood glucose. If this is more than 3 mmol/l you will just have to let him rest.

37 My teenage son refuses to take extra carbohydrate when he is hypo and insists that we let him sleep it off. Is this all right?

Hypos should always be corrected as quickly as possible. Your son is right in thinking that the insulin will eventually wear off and his blood glucose will return to normal. However, if the blood glucose falls to very low levels it could cause problems and he may even become unconscious. His refusal to take sugar is part of the confusion that occurs during a hypo and if he can be persuaded to take glucose he will get better more quickly.

38 *I have been diabetic on insulin for 38 years and my hypos have always been mild. Recently I suffered two black-outs lasting a minute which I presume were hypos. Why has this started?*

Black-outs are more common in children who have not yet learned to recognize the warning signs of a hypo. Sometimes as people get older the 'adrenaline' warnings of hypo (p.34) may fail to operate. This failure may be due to the natural ageing process or to diabetic damage to the involuntary nerve supply or may occur if the blood glucose falls very rapidly.

39 *My father has been a diabetic for 20 years. Recently he has had what his doctor calls epileptic fits. Would you tell me how to help him and if there is a cure?*

A bad hypo may bring on an epileptic fit and it is important to check your father's blood glucose during an attack. If it is low then reducing his insulin should stop the fits. If his epilepsy is not related to diabetes then it should be quite easy to control by taking tablets regularly.

40 *Can insulin reactions eventually cause permanent brain damage?*

This question is often asked and is a great source of anxiety to diabetics. The brain quickly recovers from a hypo and there is no permanent damage, even after a severe attack with convulsions. Very prolonged hypoglycaemia can occur in a patient with a tumour that produces insulin and if someone is unconscious for days on end then the brain will not recover completely. This does not occur in diabetics, in whom the insulin wears off after a few hours.

41 *I have heard that there is an opposite to insulin called glucagon. Is this something like glucose and can it be used to bring a diabetic round from a hypo?*

Glucagon is a hormone which like insulin is produced by the pancreas. Glucagon causes release into the bloodstream of glucose from stores of starch in the liver. It can be used to bring a diabetic round from a hypo though it is not often needed as sugar does the same job a great deal more cheaply. However, if a diabetic is unconscious in a hypo it may be impossible to get him to swallow glucose. Under these circumstances, glucagon given by injection may be used. The usual dose is 1 mg given into a muscle — though an ordinary subcutaneous injection will do (*see* Plate 2). Recently a smaller dose has been recommended — half the ampoule is usually effective. When the patient comes round it is best to give him some sugar as glucagon may only have a short-term effect.

42 *Is it normal to vomit shortly after a glucagon injection?*

Some people do vomit after regaining consciousness after a glucagon injection, particularly children. If only half the contents of the ampoule is given, it will usually be enough to correct the hypo, but is less likely to cause sickness.

43 *Since I have been put on one of the new purified insulins I never know when I am going hypo. Several other people in the clinic have also noticed this. Is this a common problem?*

Several diabetics have reported this finding though it is not easy to find an explanation for it. Purified insulins should not have any different action from the old insulin. The *rate* at which the blood glucose falls may alter the way people feel when they are going hypo. Purified insulin may be absorbed more rapidly and so bring down the blood glucose more quickly thus altering the warning signs of a hypo. Most people who change to new insulins seem to get used to them in a few weeks.

44 *My diabetes was controlled by tablets for 20 years but two years ago my doctor recommended that I begin insulin treatment. I am well controlled but my sleep is often disturbed by dreams — or I wake up feeling hungry. Can you advise me what to do if this happens?*

It sounds as though you are going hypo in the middle of the night. It has been shown that many diabetics have a low blood glucose in the early hours of the night and provided they feel all right and sleep well this probably does not matter. However, if you are regularly waking with hypo symptoms (such as hunger) or having nightmares you should first check that you are hypo by measuring your blood glucose at around 3.00 a.m. If the reading is low you need to reduce the evening dose of medium-acting insulin. If the blood glucose is then high before breakfast the next day, an injection of medium-acting insulin before going to bed may solve the problem.

45 *What can I do if my diabetic son has a bad hypo and is too drowsy to take any glucose by mouth?*

First try giving him some strong glucose (or sugar) containing solution to sip — Lucozade may be helpful here or some people try a spoonful of honey or ordinary jam. Fluids should not be given by mouth if he is unconscious. If he will not take any by mouth, there are two alternatives — either an injection of sterile glucose into a vein or else an injection of glucagon (p.37) under the skin, like insulin. Injecting glucose into a vein can be difficult and can usually only be done by a doctor. Glucagon is much easier to inject but has the disadvantage that it may cause vomiting.

46 *Am I correct in thinking that only diabetics on insulin can have hypos?*

No. Some of the tablets used for diabetes cause hypos. The commonly used ones are glibenclamide (Euglucon, Daonil) and chlorpropamide (Diabenese). These hypos will improve with glucose in the normal way but because the tablets have a longer action than insulin the hypo may return again for several hours.

Chlorpropamide is particularly dangerous in this respect as the hypos may have an effect for 36 hours. Anyone having hypos on tablets probably needs to reduce the dose. Metformin does not cause hypos.

47 *I am a diabetic on diet alone and have headaches and a light-headed feeling around midday if I have been busy in the morning. I am all right after eating something. Why is this?*

It seems surprising but some mild diabetics can go hypo if they go without food. This is because they produce their own insulin but too late and sometimes too much. You should check that you are hypo by measuring blood glucose at a time when you feel odd. If you are hypo you will be able to avoid this by eating snacks between meals.

48 *My daughter aged 21 is a diabetic on insulin and is moving down to London where she hopes to rent a flat on her own. In view of the risk of hypoglycaemic attacks, would you advise against this?*

By the age of 21 your daughter should be quite capable of looking after herself and this includes living in a flat by herself — in London or anywhere else for that matter. There is no need to worry about hypos at night as the insulin will wear off in due course and no serious harm can occur. The only time when hypos are potentially dangerous are during such activities as driving and swimming.

If your daughter is sensible she will tell close friends and workmates that she is diabetic and explain that she must be given sugar if she behaves oddly. Diabetics often fail to take this simple precaution which can avoid a lot of worry to their friends who may find them hypo and yet have no idea how to help.

Practical aspects

49 *When I was discharged from hospital as a new insulin-dependent diabetic I was given a few disposable syringes and needles for my injections. However, when I went to my own GP to get more supplies he told me I could only have a glass syringe with metal needles. Was he correct?*

Yes, I am afraid he was. At the present time the only insulin syringes and needles that are available free to diabetics from their own GPs on prescription are glass syringes and stainless-steel reusable needles. Equipment for injections that is available free on the 'drug tariff' as it is called are BS 1619/2 glass syringes, a plastic syringe carrying case, a pack of reusable stainless-steel needles, and industrial methylated spirit for keeping the syringe and needle clean in the syringe carrying case. If you are using glass syringes you should always have a spare syringe in case one breaks and if this happens immediately replace the spare by asking your GP for a new prescription. In Scotland disposable needles are available for all under the age of 16 years via the Health Board.

50 *Whilst drawing up my insulin my glass syringe cracked. As I did not have a spare I gave the injection as best I could but lost some of the insulin. Will this do any harm?*

If you lost much insulin your blood glucose results or urine tests would probably be higher than normal during the day. Always make sure you have a spare glass syringe at home.

51 *What is the best way of sterilizing glass syringes? I have boiled them for many years but my hospital clinic have said that method is out of date*

We do not recommend that you boil glass syringes as they crack and break easily after being boiled several times. It is also rather time consuming and the syringes wear out more quickly as a result of 'scale' accummulating on the syringe from the boiled water. The most common method these days is to store the glass syringe (and needle) in a syringe carrying case that is half-filled with industrial methylated spirit (*not* surgical spirit) and change the spirit in the case about once a week. Before drawing up the insulin the plunger should be worked up and down several times to get rid of the spirit.

52 *I have recently been told that I should not use surgical spirit for keeping my glass syringe sterile. Why is this?*

Surgical spirit contains an oily base and makes the syringe slippery to hold. It also makes the plunger jam in the syringe. Many diabetics who have used surgical spirit in the past rinsed their syringes in boiling water or under the tap to get rid of the surgical spirit but we do not recommend this as it makes the injection more time consuming and it is difficult to remove the oily substance. If you are keeping your glass syringe in spirit this should be 70% industrial methylated spirit (IMS) which is colourless and can be obtained only on prescription. Ordinary methylated spirit has a dye added to it and is also unsuitable for use.

53 *I have recently heard that disposable syringes and needles can be reused. How many times can they be reused and how can they be kept clean in between injections?*

Although the manufacturers state that disposable syringes and needles are for 'single use only', we recommend that they may be reused. Plastic or disposable syringes that come with a *detachable* needle can be used for several weeks. Most plastic syringes will not last much longer than a couple of weeks because either the marks start to wear off or the plunger becomes sticky and difficult to push up and down. Disposable needles can be reused until the needle becomes blunt. For some people this may be 2 days, for others it may be 2 weeks. Many people find they can use them longer and more comfortably than they can a regular steel needle. The most commonly used U100 syringes come complete with a fixed needle on the end of the syringe and therefore this will last only as long as the needle. We do not recommend that syringes with fixed needles are used for more than half a dozen injections as the needles *may* have a tendency to break. Some 'cloudy' insulins have a tendency to clog the fine-gauge needles when reused too frequently.

Disposable syringes should be kept dry between injections, preferably in a clean place specially reserved in a normal domestic fridge. They must never be boiled and should not be kept in any type of spirit as the marks come off.

Disposable needles used with disposable syringes can be left on the end of the plastic syringe with the protective cover carefully replaced over the needle and left together with the syringe in the fridge. Monoject syringes can be replaced in their original casing and an extended cap is available to protect the protruding plunger of pre-filled syringes. Disposable (plastic hub) needles used with glass syringes can be left on the end of the syringe in the spirit proof carrying case. They can be safely kept in industrial methylated spirit without the protective cover on the end.

54 *I understand that I am unable to obtain disposable syringes and needles on prescription from my GP, but can I buy these from a chemist without a prescription?*

Yes. If you are not being given disposable syringes and needles by your hospital clinic you can obtain them at little cost, without prescription, at your local chemist or you can take advantage of the excellent postal service offered by Mariner Medical Ltd, Hypoguard Ltd or Owen Mumford Ltd (*see* Appendix 2).

55 *There is a bewildering array of syringes and needles on the market. Which are the best types to use?*

Since the introduction of U100 insulin, if glass syringes are prescribed these must be either the 0.5 ml (millilitre) syringe marked with 50 single divisions for those diabetics taking not more than 50 units of insulin in one injection or the 1 ml (millilitre) syringe marked up to 100 units in 2-unit divisions for those diabetics taking more than 50 units of insulin in one injection.

These syringes are known as BS 1619/2 and should be marked with the word INSULIN on the side of the syringe. Similar syringes are available in the disposable variety either with a detachable needle or a fixed needle. They come in either $\frac{1}{2}$ ml (0.5 ml) or 1 ml sizes and are correspondingly marked with either 50 or 100 unit divisions (Figure 1). They also have the word INSULIN marked on the side. Insulin must never be drawn up into a syringe that is not marked in this way.

Some people prefer to use syringes that come with a detachable needle as they can reuse the syringe more economically whilst others prefer the neat packaging and the fine-gauge needles of the syringe–needle combinations such as B-D plastipak or Monoject.

Disposable syringes and needles are listed at the end of this section and *see* Plate 7.

56 What is the best size of needle to use for an insulin injection?

Needles come in a variety of gauges and lengths. The gauge or G refers to wire gauge; the lower the number, the thicker the 'wire' the needle is made from. Most people prefer to use the finest possible needle which is known as the 'fine gauge' needle and comes as a 27.5G or 28G needle. The 1/2 (half inch) refers to the length of the needle and is the length of choice for most diabetics. Some very thin people may prefer a three-eighths (3/8ths) needle whilst fatter people may use a five-eighths (5/8ths) needle. We do not recommend anything longer than five-eighths of an inch or thicker than 26G.

57 What syringes are available for the blind or poorly sighted diabetic?

There is a pre-set syringe which has an adjustable locking nut on the syringe plunger which can be altered by a sighted person so that the plunger can only be drawn back to a certain point. The disadvantage with this syringe is that this nut can move out of place unless screwed up very tightly and

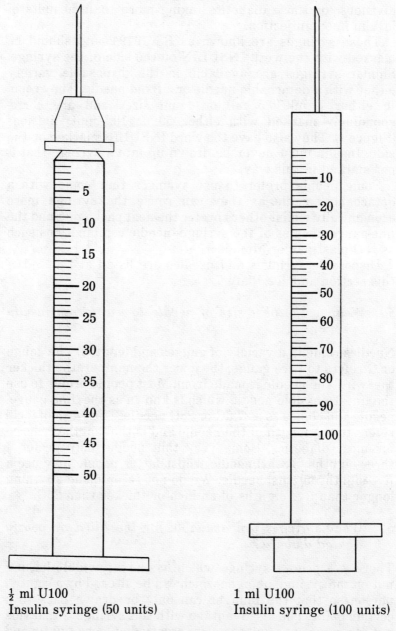

½ ml U100
Insulin syringe (50 units)

1 ml U100
Insulin syringe (100 units)

Figure 1   Insulin syringes for ½ ml U100 and 1 ml U100.

then the wrong amount of insulin will be drawn up. It is also impossible to mix two types of insulin in the same syringe. This syringe is available on prescription from your GP.

A much more practical syringe is the Click/Count syringe which is made by Hypoguard Ltd. This syringe 'clicks' for every mark on the syringe and has two positions, a free position where the plunger moves freely up and down and a clicking position where the plunger clicks into place for every mark. The positions can be changed by turning the plunger a quarter-turn clockwise. Although it may take a little time to get used to the syringe, with practice there is little chance of error, and two types of insulin can be drawn into the same syringe. With the introduction of 100 u/ml insulin the U100 Click/Count syringe is also available on prescription from your GP. The U100 Click/Count syringe is only available in a 1 ml size and therefore one click on the syringe is equal to two units of insulin.

Two useful pieces of equipment to be used with either the pre-set or Click/Count syringe are a location tray that lines up the syringe/needle and insulin bottle or the Centre Point Needle Guide. These are also obtainable from Hypoguard Ltd.

Becton-Dickinson, Sherwood and Mariner Medical (Mariner is the Monoject Diabetic Consumer Unit) can supply magnifiers which clip over their plastic syringes which may make the marks easier to read. Rand Rocket produce, free of charge, a plastic gauge for use with 1 ml Terumo syringes (ABCare) (*see* Plate 9).

58　*My son has trouble giving himself injections and has asked me if he can use an injector. What type of injector should he use?*

With modern syringes and fine-gauge disposable needles injections are rarely a problem if the correct technique is used (Plate 3). Most people find injectors more trouble than they are worth and are something extra to carry around. The most commonly used injector in this country is the Hypoguard injector which is easy to use. However, care must be taken when using the Hypoguard with a mixture of insulins to ensure that the insulins are always drawn up in the same order every time as there is a large 'dead space' in the injector which may cause variation in the insulin dose when two insulins are mixed together. This injector is also available for use with B-D Plastipak Lo-Dose 1/2 ml and 1 ml syringes which eliminates the problem of 'dead space'. Its main advantage is that it prevents you from seeing the needle when the injection is given. Another injector is the Palmer Gun which is gripped like a pistol and is sometimes preferred by children although it is bulky. One of the better injectors is the Busher injector which is made by Becton-Dickinson in the USA and was originally designed for their glass syringes. It now comes with a plastic device that enables it to be used with B-D Plastipak 1 ml syringes but can be difficult to obtain in the UK. Another aid for injection which may be useful for people who take multiple daily injection is the Button Infuser. This is a small button shaped plastic item about the size and weight of a one pence piece. When its fine needle is inserted the button is anchored flat against the skin with a small adhesive pad and, once in place, insulin can be injected into the button's needle target which has a reusable cap. It is available from Rand Rocket Ltd.

The Hypoguard Injector may be obtained from Hypoguard Ltd (*see* Appendix 2).

The Palmer Gun may be obtained from Palmer Injectors Ltd, 11 George Square, Glasgow G2 1EA.

Enquiries about the Busher Injector should be sent to Becton-Dickinson UK Ltd, Between Towns Road, Cowley, Oxford OX4 3LY.

59 What is the 'jet' injector?

This is an injector which works by firing liquid, such as insulin, through the skin from very high pressure jets. It is not entirely painless, is very bulky, very expensive, unsuitable for those who mix insulins and has not yet been proved to be harmless when multiple injections are given, i.e. by a diabetic giving twice daily insulin for several years. Until more is known about the long-term effects we would not advise its use.

60 Is it necessary to use spirit before or after injecting myself?

To reduce the chance of transferring infection from one patient to another, doctors and nurses swab the skin with spirit (alcohol) when giving injections in hospital. For a long time diabetics were taught to do the same but it is now realized that it is unnecessary as infection is unlikely to be introduced from normal skin. We advise against the use of spirit as it tends to harden the skin. If you feel you must clean the injection site (say after playing football) use soap and water only.

61 Is it dangerous to inject air bubbles that may be in the syringe after drawing up insulin?

The only reason you are taught to get rid of large air bubbles from the syringe after drawing up insulin is because the air takes the place of the insulin and therefore the dose will not be accurate. *Very large* quantities of air injected directly into the circulation can be dangerous by producing an air lock in the bloodstream but these amounts are far larger than could possibly be introduced when injecting insulin. Tiny air bubbles, even when introduced into a vein, would not do any harm and would quickly be absorbed.

62 Can two types of insulin be mixed in the same syringe?

Yes, many patients these days are taking mixtures of insulin. Unless instructed otherwise by your doctor you should inject mixtures of insulin immediately after they are drawn up.

The rule when drawing up two types of insulin is to draw up the clear (short-acting) insulin first followed by the cloudy (longer-acting) insulin. The reason for this is to prevent the clear bottle of insulin becoming 'contaminated' by the cloudy insulin. If this happens the clear or short-acting insulin loses its quick-acting properties. The correct way of mixing insulins in the same syringe is illustrated in Plate 5.

63   When drawing up my insulin I sometimes find that the insulin gets 'sucked back' into the bottle. Why is this?

This is due to not putting air into the bottle before drawing up the insulin. You should inject the same volume of air into the bottle as the amount of insulin you intend to draw out. If you do not do this a vacuum will develop and either the insulin will be sucked back into the bottle or it will be difficult to get the insulin out. So remember to prime the bottle with air from your syringe before trying to draw up insulin (*see* Plate 4).

64   I have been giving my insulin injections at an angle of about 45 degrees for many years but have recently been told that this is incorrect. What do you advise?

In the past diabetics were taught to pinch up the skin and then inject at an angle of 45 degrees. One of the problems with this method has been that the depth of the injection could be very variable depending on the length of the needle or how much the angle of injection varied. Insulin is designed to be given into the deep layer of fat under the skin and with a shallow angle of injection the insulin often is not given deep enough. Diabetics are now taught to use a 26–28G half-inch needle and to give the injection at right angles to the skin without pinching the skin up first. This encourages the injection to be given more quickly which means that it should be virtually painless. If you experience difficulty pushing the needle through the skin it can often be helpful to stretch the skin between finger and thumb so that it is less likely to 'resist' the needle. If you prefer to give the injection by first pinching up the skin always pick up a generous portion of fat and do not squeeze too tightly as this may cause bruising. The needle should still be pushed in quickly at virtually right angles to the skin. See illustrations in Plate 3 for correct methods of injection technique.

65 *My young daughter spends a very long time giving her injection and complains that it is painful. Is there any advice you can give?*

One of the reasons that she finds it painful is because she is probably pushing the needle slowly through the skin. The sensitive nerve endings lie virtually on the surface of the skin and are more likely to be stimulated if the needle enters the skin very slowly. Try to encourage her to push the needle through the skin as quickly as possible. The use of disposable 'microfine' 27G half-inch needles will also make things easier. If she still experiences difficulty then the ice-cube technique may be helpful. A cube of ice can be held against the skin for about 10 seconds which 'freezes' the skin just long enough for the injection to be given. This method can be employed until confidence has been gained with the giving of injections.

66 *Sometimes after giving my injection I find that a small lump appears just under the skin. What is the cause of this?*

It sounds as though you are giving the injection at too shallow a depth. If the insulin is injected just below the skin (intradermal) a small lump will appear. Apart from being more painful the insulin will not be absorbed properly. Try giving the injection more deeply by injecting at right angles to the skin (*see* Plate 3) and this will not happen.

67 *Should I draw back on the plunger after inserting the needle to check for blood?*

It used to be common practice to teach diabetics to draw back on the plunger before injecting insulin to check that the needle had not entered a blood vessel. These days we are less inclined to teach this as the chances of insulin entering a blood vessel are extremely slight and pulling back on the plunger may make the injection more difficult for some people. If you are in the habit of drawing back before giving insulin by all means continue but it is not strictly necessary.

68   Sometimes after giving my injection I notice that the injection site bleeds a lot. Does this do any harm?

This may happen if you puncture a blood capillary (very small blood vessel) which means that the needle goes straight through the capillary. This usually means that the injection site will bleed rather heavily and you will probably see a bruise there the following day, but it does no harm.

69   When I have given my injection I sometimes see some insulin leaking out from the injection hole after taking out the needle. Should I give myself extra insulin later and how much should I give?

Insulin does sometimes leak out immediately after having given the injection and this can often be avoided by moving the skin to one side immediately after withdrawing the needle or alternatively moving the skin to one side *before inserting* the needle. This effectively means that the needle channel closes after the needle has been withdrawn. If either of these methods fail then have a tissue handy at injection time ready to press straight on the spot after giving the injection. Extra insulin should not be given if you lose a little because you will not know how much has been lost and will probably over-compensate, give too much and risk hypoglycaemia. Having taken too little insulin may mean that your urine tests or blood sugar levels will be just higher than normal that day.

70   The layer of fat beneath the surface of the skin of my thighs is very hard and I find it difficult to inject myself. Have you any suggestions?

This could be due to not rotating injection sites and re-using the same place too many times which causes the flesh to become hard and as a result leads to erratic absorption of the insulin. These over-used areas should not be injected for about a year and new areas found. Another possible cause for hard skin is the use of spirit for swabbing the skin which makes the skin tough and difficult to inject. Stop swabbing the skin (p.47) and try softening it by rubbing in hand cream

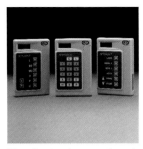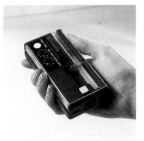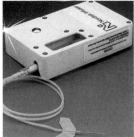

Plate 1   A selection of insulin pumps (from left to right CPI, Graseby, Nordisk).

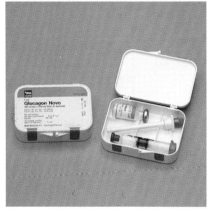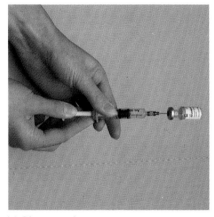

Plate 2   a) 1 mg of glucagon.

b) Glucagon drawn into syringe prior to administration.

Plate 3   How to inject

Method one

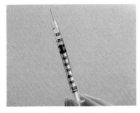

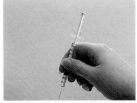

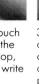

1. Make absolutely certain once again that you have measured your insulin dose to the correct mark on the syringe.

2. Taking care not to touch the sterile needle, hold the syringe firmly near the top, as if you were going to write with it like a pencil.

3. Now, using the thumb and the forefinger of the other hand, stretch flat an area of clear skin and quickly push the needle straight in as far as it will go.

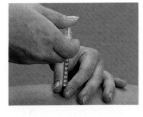

4. Hold the syringe barrel comfortably in place with one hand so that your other hand is free to press the plunger. With your thumb on top of the plunger, quickly and smoothly inject all of the insulin in the syringe.

5. Withdraw the needle and quickly place a clean piece of tissue or cotton wool over the injection site. Hold it in place with firm pressure for just a few seconds. Your injection is completed.

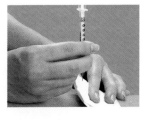

Method two

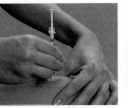

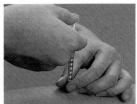

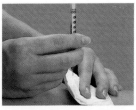

1. Hold the syringe like a pencil, as if you were going to write with it. Now, using the other hand, pinch up a mound of clean skin and quickly push the needle straight into the mound as far as it will go. (Some people prefer to insert the needle at a slight angle—almost vertical but not quite.)

2. Release the mound of skin. Hold the syringe barrel comfortably in place with one hand so that your other hand is free to press the plunger.
With your thumb on top of the plunger, quickly and smoothly inject all of the insulin in the syringe.

3. Withdraw the needle and quickly place a clean piece of tissue or cotton wool over the injection site. Hold it in place with firm pressure for just a few seconds. Your injection is completed.

Plate 4　One dose injection

Here is the step-by-step routine for measuring your insulin from one bottle

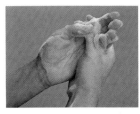

1. Wash your hands and dry them.

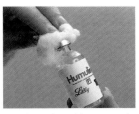

2. Clean the rubber cap of the bottle with cotton wool and industrial spirit or with a single-use alcohol swab.

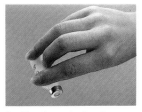

3. Gently tip the bottle to and fro to make sure that the insulin is properly mixed. This is especially important when using cloudy insulin.

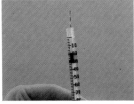

4. Pull back the plunger of the syringe to measure approx. the same amount of air as the amount of insulin you use.

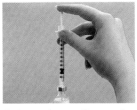

5. Insert the needle straight through the rubber cap of the insulin bottle and inject the air into the bottle.

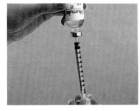

6. Now turn the bottle upside down. Make certain that the point of the needle inside the bottle is well beneath the surface level of the insulin.

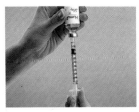

7. Continue holding the bottle and syringe upright with the point upwards and pull back the plunger until you have measured slightly more than your correct dose of insulin.

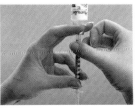

8. If any air bubbles have entered the syringe, tap the syringe barrel fairly gently with your finger and this will usually release them so that they rise to the tip of the syringe.
NOTE: If the air bubbles persist, expel all of the insulin back into the bottle and start again.

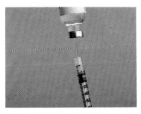

9. Press the plunger slightly to expel the bubbles back into the bottle. Adjust the plunger to measure your exact insulin dose and take the needle out of the bottle.

Plate 5   Mixed dose injection

If you use two types of insulin for a mixed dose then this is the way to do it

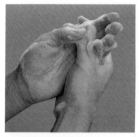

1. Wash your hands and dry them.

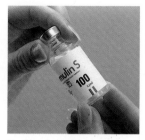

2. Check the labels on the insulin bottles for any special instructions.

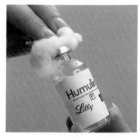

3. Clean the rubber caps of the bottles with cotton wool and industrial spirit or with a single-use alcohol swab.

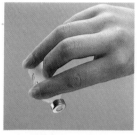

4. Gently tip each bottle to and fro to make sure that the insulin is properly mixed. This is especially important for the cloudy insulins.

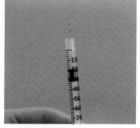

5. Pull back the plunger of the syringe to measure approx. the same amount of air as the amount of cloudy insulin that you use.

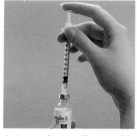

6. Insert the needle straight through the rubber cap of the cloudy insulin bottle and inject the air into the bottle.

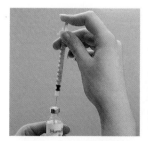

6a. Keep the plunger fully pressed down and remove the needle from the bottle.

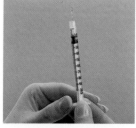

7. Pull back the plunger of the syringe to measure approx. the same amount of air as the amount of clear insulin that you use.

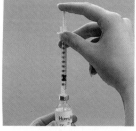

8. Insert the needle straight through the rubber cap of the clear insulin bottle and inject the air into the bottle.

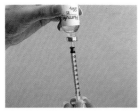

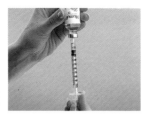

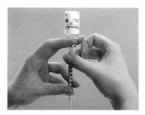

9. Now turn the bottle upside down. Make certain that the point of the needle inside the bottle is well beneath the surface level of the insulin.

10. Continue holding the bottle and syringe upright with the point upwards and pull back the plunger until you have measured slightly more than your correct dose of clear insulin.

11. If any air bubbles have entered the syringe, tap the syringe barrel fairly gently with your finger and this will usually release them so that they rise to the tip of the syringe.
NOTE: If any air bubbles persist, expel all of the clear insulin back into the bottle and start again.

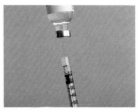

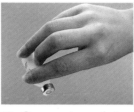

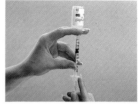

12. Press the plunger slightly to expel the bubbles back into the bottle. Adjust the plunger to measure your exact dose of clear insulin. Withdraw the needle from the bottle.

13. Once again, gently tip the cloudy insulin bottle to and fro to make sure that the insulin is properly mixed.

14. Now re-insert the needle into the upturned bottle of cloudy insulin. Make certain that the point of the needle inside the bottle is well beneath the surface level of the insulin. Carefully pull back the plunger until you have measured your exact dose of cloudy insulin.

14a. **Very important** If you accidentally measure too much cloudy insulin DO NOT press the plunger and return the excess amount into the bottle because some clear insulin will also be injected into the cloudy insulin bottle. Just remove the needle from the bottle, press the plunger to the bottom and discharge all of the insulin from the syringe into the sink. Then start again from 5.

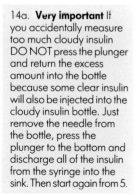

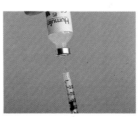

15a **Very important**
Always measure your two insulins in the same order every day.

15. Withdraw the needle from the cloudy bottle.

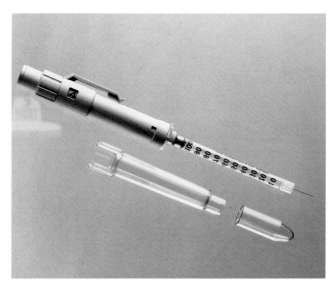

Plate 6   The Penject by Hypoguard Ltd.

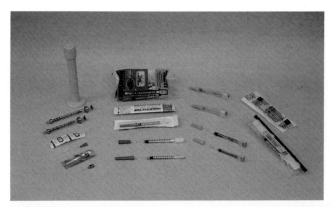

Plate 7   A selection of U100 insulin syringes and needles. (From left to right glass syringes and carrying case, BD Plastipak, Monoject, Sabre and Terumo.)

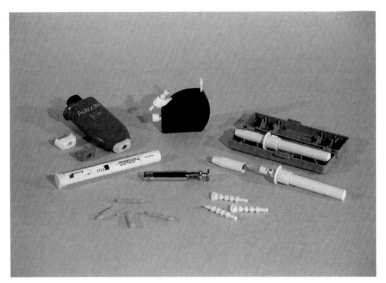

Plate 8 A selection of finger prickers (from left to right back – Autoclix, Autolet, Autolancet (in box) middle – Monojector, Hypoguard Autolancet (out of box) front – Unilet and Monolet blood lancets.

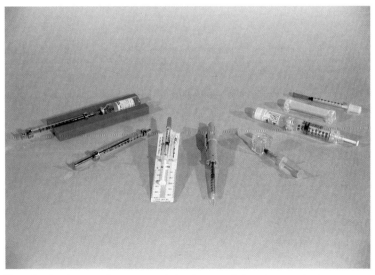

Plate 9 A selection of injection aids for the visually handicapped. (From left to right click/count syringe and location tray—click/count syringe. ABCare gauge and syringe. Penject, Monoject magnifier, and BD plastipak magnifiers.)

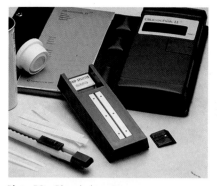

Plate 10 Blood glucose meters
a) Glucochek II and strip splitter.

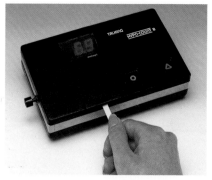

b) Talking Hypocount (for the visually handicapped)

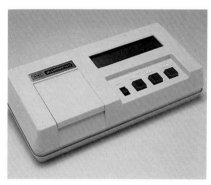

c) Ames Glucometer

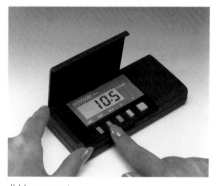

d) Hypocount

at night. If the needle still appears to be resisted by the skin try stretching the skin before injecting at right angles.

71 I have been taking insulin for 18 years and have unsightly bulges at the top of my thighs where I give my injections. How can I get rid of them?

These bulges which are known as lipohypertrophy are due to the build-up of fat below the skin. This is almost certainly caused by constantly injecting insulin into the same site over several years. Insulin will not be absorbed properly from these areas and the sites should not be used for at least a year. We would suggest that you do not use the top of your thighs at all for a couple of years. Inject into your abdomen or buttocks over the next few months, and then rotate to your upper arms for a few months. Then return to the buttocks or abdomen until the thighs have been 'rested'. When you return to the thighs use a much larger area than you have previously used, and try to avoid the top of the thighs.

72 Where is the best place to give an injection of insulin?

Insulin is designed to be given into the deep layers of fat below the skin and basically can be given in any place where there is a reasonable layer of fat. The recommended places are the fronts and sides of the middle or upper thighs, the abdomen and the buttocks. The upper arms may also be used, but some women prefer not to use the arms in the summer months in case they have marks at the injection sites which may be noticeable when wearing summer dresses. The calf can also be used and may be helpful for men if they are injecting away from home as they only need to lift up a trouser leg to give the injection. It is very important not to develop 'favourite' injection areas, and to change to new sites regularly. Suitable sites for injection are shown in Figure 2.

Figure 2
Suitable sites for
insulin injection.

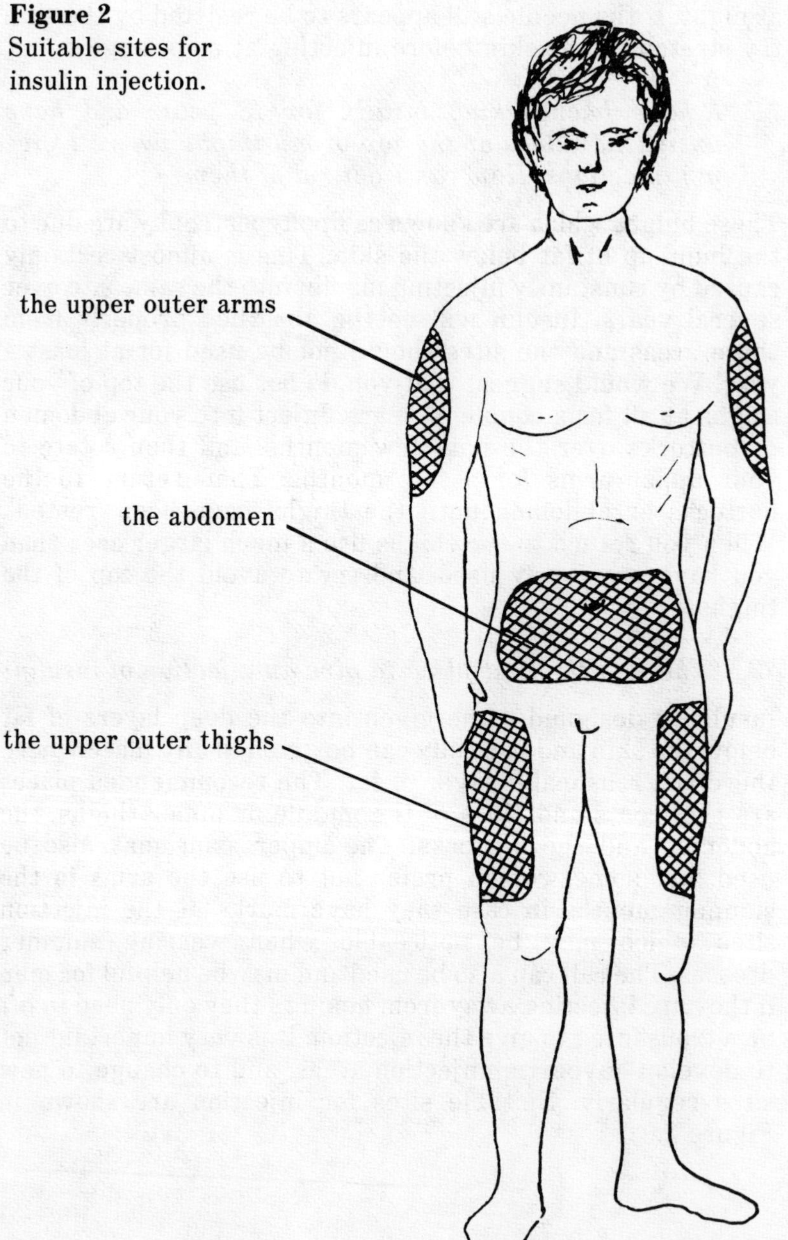

the upper outer arms

the abdomen

the upper outer thighs

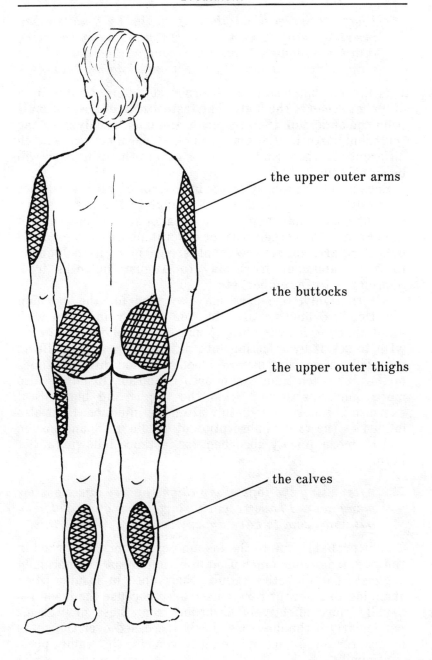

the upper outer arms

the buttocks

the upper outer thighs

the calves

73 I have to increase my dose of insulin by 4 units when injecting into my arms and by 6 units when injecting into the abdomen to maintain control. Can you tell me why this is, and should I inject only into my thighs?

It is known that insulin is absorbed at different rates from different areas of the body. The fastest rate of absorption is from the abdomen, then the arms and most slowly from the thigh and buttocks. For many people this will not make much difference to their control but for others the difference will be significant.

Because of this known factor in absorption rates we do not normally suggest that diabetics change to a new site every day but rather that they use one area for several months and then change to another area for several months and followed by a third area for several months, e.g. thighs from January to April, abdomen from May to August, buttocks from September to December, etc.

Alternatively, one area may be used for the morning injection and another area for the evening injection with some changes if away from home or on holiday. You may wish to see if by injecting into different areas this affects control by measuring several blood sugars at different times of the day, each time a new area is chosen. Insulin is also more quickly absorbed from the thighs and buttocks if exercise is taken immediately after the injection. Heat also influences the rate of absorption of insulin (p.28) and insulin will be more quickly absorbed, for instance following a hot bath.

74 After using the tops of my thighs for my injections for many years I have recently started using my abdomen but now seem to have hypos every day. Why is this?

This is probably due to the insulin being poorly absorbed in the past from your much-used injection areas. We normally suggest that diabetics reduce their dose of insulin when changing to a new or rarely used area because the insulin is usually more effectively absorbed from these new areas, particularly if the dose has slowly increased over the years owing to the injection being given in the same place continually.

75   Where should I keep my supplies of insulin?

Stores of insulin should ideally be kept in a refrigerator *not* in the freezer or freezing compartment. The best place is the vegetable compartment, or the door of the fridge which will ensure that there is no possibility of the insulin freezing. If you do not have a fridge, insulin will retain its strength for over a year if kept away from direct heat (such as radiators and direct sunlight). The insulin bottle that you have in current use should be kept at room temperature as insulin is more comfortable to give if it is not used straight from the fridge.

76   I have large hollows on my arms and legs where I give my insulin injections. What are these and can I get rid of them?

These hollows are known as lipoatrophy and are due to the disappearance of fat from beneath the skin. It is not serious but does not look very attractive and can almost certainly be cured by changing to highly purified insulin (p.22).

77   What is a Penject?

Penject is a device which is used with a Becton Dickinson U100 1 ml syringe. Using the Penject, insulin is drawn into the syringe until full so that it becomes a 'cartridge' of insulin and can be conveniently carried around in a pocket or handbag without the need to carry an insulin bottle. Injections consist of simply selecting the amount of insulin to be injected by adjusting the rotating selection ring, inserting the needle and pressing the delivery button. The injection relies on normal finger pressure, i.e. it is not a 'gun'. It cannot be used by people who are taking certain mixtures of insulin but is very useful for people who take multiple injections of insulin. It is obtainable from Hypoguard Ltd (*see* Plate 6).

78   Should I wipe the top of the insulin bottle with spirit before drawing up the required dose?

Although many clinics teach people to clean the tops of the insulin bottles, we do not think that it is necessary.

See Plate 7 for a selection of U 100 insulin syringes and needles.

Disposable U 100 syringes with fixed needles

Monoject: $\frac{1}{2}$ ml syringe with fixed 27G × $\frac{1}{2}$″ needle

Monoject: 1 ml syringe with fixed 27G × $\frac{1}{2}$″ needle

B D Plastipak: Lo-Dose $\frac{1}{2}$ ml syringe with fixed 28G × $\frac{1}{2}$″ needle

B D Plastipak: 1 ml syringe with fixed 28G × $\frac{1}{2}$″ needle

ABCare (Terumo): 1 ml syringe with fixed 27.5G × $\frac{1}{2}$″ needle

Disposable U 100 syringes with detachable needles

Steriseal: 1 ml syringe with 27G × $\frac{5}{8}$″ needle

Steriseal: 1 ml syringe with 25G × $\frac{5}{8}$″ needle

ABCare (Terumo): 1 ml syringe with 26G × $\frac{1}{2}$″ needle

Gillette: 1 ml syringe with 25G × $\frac{5}{8}$″ needle

Disposable U 100 syringe without needle

Gillette: 1 ml syringe

Steriseal: 1 ml syringe

ABCare: 1 ml syringe

Disposable needles

Becton Dickinson: 26G × $\frac{1}{2}$″

Becton Dickinson: 25G × $\frac{5}{8}$″

Monoject: 27G × $\frac{1}{2}$″

Monoject: 25G × $\frac{5}{8}$″

ABCare: 26G × $\frac{1}{2}$″

ABCare: 27G × $\frac{3}{4}$″

Gillette: 25G × $\frac{5}{8}$″

ABCare: 25G × $\frac{5}{8}$″

NB: The authors recommend the use of 26G, 27G, 27.5G or 28G × $\frac{1}{2}$″ needle used with either a separate syringe or as a syringe–needle combination. This length needle should be injected at right angles to the skin (p.48). Syringe–needle combinations, such as Monoject or B D

Plastipak, are perhaps the most convenient syringes. Most of these syringes and needles can be obtained from either Hypoguard or Owen Mumford, or local chemists. Monoject syringes are also obtainable from Mariner Medical. ABCare syringes are also obtainable from Rand Rocket.

Tablets

79 I understand that there are two different sorts of 'diabetic' tablets. Can you tell me what they are and what the difference is between them?

The two different groups of tablets which may be used for certain diabetics are (a) sulphonylureas which include chlorpropamide (Diabinese), glibenclamide (Daonil, Euglucon) and tolbutamide (Rastinon) and (b) biguanides — e.g. metformin (Glucophage). The two groups of drugs work in different ways. Sulphonylureas act mainly by increasing the amount of natural insulin from the pancreas; biguanides on the other hand increase the uptake of glucose by muscle and also reduce absorption of glucose by the intestine. Tablets are only effective when a reasonable amount of natural insulin is produced, so they cannot be used in most young diabetics where the pancreas makes minimal amounts of insulin or even no insulin at all.

Tablets should always be used in conjunction with a diet restricting sugars. In elderly, overweight diabetics the first line of treatment is generally diet and tablets should be kept in reserve. The sulphonylurea group of tablets have a tendency to cause further weight increase.

80 My doctor has recently asked me to stop taking phenformin and I have heard of this happening to other diabetics. Why is this?

Phenformin (Dibotin) often causes an increase in blood levels of lactic acid, which is normally present only in minute quantities. In very rare cases this level can reach danger point and cause the serious condition of lactic acidosis. Now that the link between phenformin and lactic acidosis has been established, this drug has been banned in many countries including UK and the USA. Metformin is in the same biguanide group of anti-diabetes tablets and may cause a slight rise in lactic acid levels, but never to a dangerous extent.

81   How long does tolbutamide remain effective? Would a tablet taken at lunch last through until high tea?

Tolbutamide tablets usually last for about 6 hours though this will vary from one person to another. It is common to take a tolbutamide tablet three times a day before each main meal or twice a day before breakfast and the main evening meal. If the last tablet is taken before lunch it would probably wear off in the night.

82   My doctor has prescribed tolbutamide which I was told should be taken before meals and followed by some carbohydrate. The label on the container states 'to be taken after meals with some liquids'. What should I do?

Tolbutamide is usually taken before meals so that it can be absorbed and have its effect just as the food arrives. In this case the chemist has got it wrong, though it probably would not make that much difference.

83   Are there 'diabetic' tablets which last longer than tolbutamide?

The two other commonly used tablets in the same group (sulphonylureas) are glibenclamide and chlorpropamide. Glibenclamide tablets act for about 18 hours and are taken once or at the most two times daily. Chlorpropamide has a very long action of 36 hours or more. For this reason it never needs to be taken more often than once a day. This long action of chlorpropamide can be dangerous in old people as if for some reason they are unable to eat, they may have a very low blood glucose level for several days.

84 Can taking too much glibenclamide cause slight dizziness?

Glibenclamide could be causing your blood glucose level to be too low and your dizziness could be a mild 'hypo' particularly if you get this feeling when taking exercise or before meals. You can easily find out by checking your blood glucose at a time that you have the dizziness. If your blood glucose level is not too low then something apart from the glibenclamide must be causing the dizziness.

85 I find I am dropping off to sleep all the time and never feel refreshed. I take 500 mg Diabinese and 500 mg metformin a day. Could I be taking too much?

Diabinese 500 mg is quite a large dose and your sleepiness *could* be due to a 'hypo'. You should check that your blood glucose is not too low (p.100). On the other hand, people with a *high* blood glucose often feel drowsy and lacking in energy. So your complaint could be due to either a low or a high blood sugar. The best way of finding out is to do a blood glucose test. There are of course other causes of dizziness which have nothing to do with diabetes!

86 My husband has had diabetes for 6 years and is taking one-and-a-half tablets of glibenclamide. He is now in his seventies and has frequent limb-twitching at night. Should he take some glucose before he goes to bed?

This limb-twitching sounds like a 'hypo'. It would be interesting to see if a few glucose tablets relieved the twitching but better still measure the blood sugar while it is going on. If the twitching is a hypo it would be better to reduce the dose of tablets rather than take extra glucose every night.

87 Can one get withdrawal symptoms when taken off Diabinese?

Some medicines, especially certain sleeping tablets and painkillers become necessary to the body if taken regularly for long periods of time. When these drugs are stopped the body reacts violently, causing withdrawal symptoms. Diabetic tablets are not like this and can be stopped quite safely — provided of course they are no longer necessary to keep the blood glucose under control. If the blood glucose begins to rise, symptoms of thirst, itching, etc., will return but they cannot be described as withdrawal symptoms.

88 *I have had a stroke and find that I cannot stop crying. Is this due to Rastinon (tolbutamide) tablets I take for my diabetes?*

Sometimes after a person has suffered a stroke he may have difficulty controlling his emotions and may laugh or cry at inappropriate times. This is nothing to do with diabetes or with the tablets you take to control it.

89 *My chemist tells me that some diabetic tablets react badly with alcohol. Can you please enlarge on this?*

A number of people who take chlorpropamide (Diabinese) experience a hot flush in the face when they drink alcohol. It seems that this flushing with chlorpropamide and alcohol runs in families and it has been used by research workers who are studying the genetics of diabetes. Fortunately none of the other anti-diabetic tablets have this effect of causing flushing with alcohol. If you are taking chlorpropamide and are troubled with the problem you could take instead an equivalent dose of glibenclamide. Alcohol may have other effects on the blood glucose in diabetics (p.171).

90 *Since taking Glucophage (metformin) I have had feelings of nausea and constant diarrhoea and have lost quite a lot of weight. Is this due to the Glucophage?*

Nausea and diarrhoea are common side-effects of Glucophage. The loss of weight could be due to poor food intake because Glucophage has reduced your appetite or else because your diabetes is out of control. Either way you should stop Glucophage or at least reduce the dose until the nausea and diarrhoea disappear. If your diabetes is then poorly controlled with high blood glucose levels (more than

10 mmol/l) you may need a different sort of tablet or perhaps
insulin injections — in addition to diet.

91 *What is the cause of the continuous metallic burning
taste in the mouth? I am 62 years of age and diabetic
controlled on tablets for the last 4 years*

You are probably taking metformin (Glucophage) tablets as
these sometimes do cause a curious taste in the mouth. If the
taste is troublesome (and it sounds pretty unpleasant) you
should stop taking metformin tablets. Other tablets for
diabetes (glibenclamide, chlorpropamide) do not cause this
side-effect.

92 *I am a diabetic controlled on tablets. My dose was
halved, and my urine was still negative to sugar. Would
it be all right to stop taking my tablets altogether to see
what happened? Obviously I should restart the tablets
if my urine showed sugar*

Your idea is probably a good one but you should also check
the blood glucose level as urine tests can sometimes be
misleading. Provided the blood glucose remains controlled
(less than 8 mmol/l) you would be better off without any
tablets. If you no longer need tablets, diet becomes even
more important for controlling your diabetes and you must
avoid putting on weight at all costs. Some people think that if
they come off tablets they are no longer diabetic but this is
not so. There is always the chance that they will need tablets
or even insulin at some stage in the future.

93 *I am 74 and on two glibenclamide tablets a day. In the
night after a very light snack my mouth goes dry. Does
this mean another tablet should be taken?*

In general thirst or a dry mouth points to poorly controlled
diabetes and it is quite common for this to be particularly
troublesome at night. You can discover if you are poorly
controlled by urine tests or blood glucose measurements. If
these tests are high and particularly if you are losing weight
and feeling rotten, then obviously you need more treatment.

This may mean better diet, more tablets or even insulin injections — and there are plenty of diabetics even at your age who do need insulin for proper control. There are of course other causes for a dry mouth at night — mouth breathing, for instance.

94 *Please tell me what is the maximum dose of tablets before insulin is required?*

People (especially diabetics) are all different and occasionally do well on high doses of tablets. In general the maximum dose of each tablet is as follows:

Group 1:
Tolbutamide (Rastinon) 500 mg — three per day
Glibenclamide (Euglucon, Daonil) 5 mg — three per day
Chlorpropamide (Diabinese) 100 mg tablets — three per day
250 mg tablets — one-and-a-half per day.

Group 2:
Metformin (Glucophage) 850 mg — two per day
500 mg — three per day.

Not more than one tablet from each group should be used at a time. Many diabetics continue to use the maximum dose of tablets for years with rather poor diabetic control (blood glucose consistently greater than 10 mmol/l). Although these people often feel *fairly well* in themselves they are usually much better off when they change to insulin. After the change to insulin people notice that they have more energy and can usually manage on a less strict diet.

95 *I am taking 2 × 100 mg Diabinese (chlorpropamide) tablets a day. Is it likely that I shall eventually require a stronger dosage or perhaps even insulin?*

A number of diabetics who take tablets do progress to needing a higher dose of tablets and sometimes eventually need insulin but it is impossible to predict which patients will 'get worse' in this way and which ones will continue for very many years remaining well controlled on a small dose of tablets.

96 *My doctor has advised me to change from tablets to insulin. Would I be right in thinking that I could avoid doing this if I cut down my intake of carbohydrate?*

No, you would probably not be right. If you are overweight you *might* be able to avoid insulin by dieting strictly and losing weight but only if you are eating more than you need at the moment. If your present food intake is the amount you need, then reducing this will only make you lose weight and in due course become weak — and you may already be suffering from thirst, weight loss and fatigue. So if you are eating too much, eat less and try to improve your control that way. If you are already dieting properly do not try to starve yourself. Accept insulin and you will probably be very grateful.

97 *My diabetes has been treated with tablets for 2 years and now my doctor has said I need insulin injections. Is my diabetes getting worse? I am very worried*

If your blood glucose can no longer be controlled with tablets, then your own pancreas is becoming less efficient in producing insulin, and in that sense your diabetes is worse. However, it does *not* mean you are going to suffer any new problems from the disease. Once you have got over the initial fear of injecting yourself (and most people manage this very quickly) then going on to insulin should not alter your life. You must certainly not worry about it and in any case you will probably feel much better.

Diet for diabetics not on insulin (NIDDM)

98 *Why do diabetics not taking insulin injections need to control their weight?*

People with non-insulin dependent diabetes (also called maturity-onset diabetes) are usually at least a little overweight. They rarely need insulin and treatment is by diet with or without tablets. In these cases, the insulin produced by the pancreas is ineffective due to the obesity (increased fat). Once the excess weight is lost this so-called insulin resistance is overcome. In addition to the control of the diabetes there are other health risks associated with obesity such as high blood pressure and heart disease which means that every effort should be made not to be overweight.

99 *Why do people put on weight?*

Your body needs energy (calories) from food and drink to fuel the body processes such as breathing which go on even when you are sleeping. Any form of physical activity such as walking, shopping, typing, etc., requires additional energy or calories. The ideal calorie or energy intake should balance the amount of energy used by the body. When this happens you will neither gain nor lose weight. If the amount of food and drink you consume provides more energy (calories) than is used in your daily activities, the extra food will be converted into body fat and you will start to put on weight. If you are overweight you need to reduce your daily intake of calories so you are eating less than your body needs so that you burn up your body fat.

100 *What are calories or joules?*

Calories or joules are a measure of the energy and heat that your body can obtain from food and drink that you consume. Although calories are commonly referred to in this country, many countries refer to joules as the measure of energy. One Calorie = 4.2 kJoules.

101 *I eat very small amounts of food and am constantly on a diet but cannot seem to lose any weight. My friend who is the same age eats four times the amount of food and remains as slim as a reed. Why is this?*

This is because your rate of metabolism is different from that of your friend. The metabolic rate is the rate at which you burn up a given amount of food. The rate depends on your own make up and although it seems unfair, some people burn up their food very fast and remain slim whilst others eat small amounts of food and put on weight easily. This metabolic rate can be altered under certain circumstances.

For example, people subjected to long periods of starvation slow their metabolic rate right down to conserve energy, whilst those who take regular, vigorous exercise speed up their rate of metabolism so they can eat more food and not put on extra weight. The only way you will lose weight is by eating less food than your body needs.

102 Do diabetics controlled by diet alone have to keep to strict mealtimes?

The need for insulin-treated diabetics to keep fairly closely to regular mealtimes is to avoid a low blood glucose (hypoglycaemia). Since diabetics treated by diet alone are not at risk from hypoglycaemia they need not keep to strict mealtimes. However, when weight reduction is important, eating small meals regularly through the day is more effective than starving for hours and then eating a very large meal.

103 Are there any appetite suppressants on the market suitable for diabetics?

Many of the 'slimming aids' on the market contain methyl cellulose, an artificial fibre which swells to a greater bulk to help fill the stomach. Although these 'slimming aids' will do no harm it is a much more sensible plan to train your stomach to expect less food at mealtimes so that you do not feel hungry and therefore reduce your calorie intake.

Appetite suppressants such as Ponderax are available only on prescription. These are generally ineffective in the long term, and are no longer widely recommended. There is no substitute for the determination to stick to a diet.

104 Is the F-Plan diet suitable for diabetics?

Yes. These days a diet for diabetics that is high in fibre (roughage) is encouraged and the F-Plan diet ensures that plenty of fibre is taken in the diet. One of the reasons that the F-Plan diet has been successful is because it is very satisfying and does not leave you feeling hungry. It is important to stress that to lose weight successfully calories need to be reduced and this means 'counting' the calories in the recipes and if necessary weighing the food used so that extra calories are not consumed.

105 *My husband's diabetes is controlled by diet alone. Since being diagnosed 2 years ago, he has kept strictly to his diet and in the past year he has not had a positive urine test and his clinic blood sugar measurements have been normal. Does this mean he is no longer diabetic?*

Once a diabetic, always a diabetic. I am afraid this applies to almost everyone and exceptions are very rare. He should be commended for keeping to his diet so well because this is the reason his diabetes is obviously so well controlled. If he went back to his old dietary habits and started putting on weight it is very likely that all the old symptoms would return and his blood sugars would be high again. It may help if his GP or local clinic continues to keep a check on him so that this successful treatment and good health can continue.

106 *Do diabetics on diet alone need to eat snacks in between meals?*

No. The reason that patients taking insulin injections are often advised to eat a snack in between their main meals is to balance the effect of the insulin they take. Patients on diet alone or diet and tablets do not have this problem and do not need the snacks. In fact if extra snacks are taken between meals this will increase the total calories taken during the day and will cause a problem with weight increase. When weight reduction is important eating small meals regularly through the day is more effective than starving for hours and then eating a single very large meal.

107 *Can I eat as much diabetic food as I like?*

No. Whether you can eat diabetic (low sugar) food depends to a large extent on your weight. If you are overweight and on a weight-reducing diet then diabetic foods (apart from diabetic fruit squash) are not suitable. Most diabetic foods and alcoholic drinks are *not* low in calories and as such cannot be fitted into the weight-reducing diet. The government recommends that these foods carry a statement about their unsuitability for the overweight on their packaging. If you are of normal weight then diabetic foods may be taken in moderation. Sorbitol which is often used as a sweetener can cause stomach upsets if taken in large quantities and the BDA recommend that fructose (another sweetener) should not be taken in larger quantities than 50 grams in weight in any one day.

108   Does sorbitol contain calories?

Yes. Sorbitol has as many calories as sugar and is therefore unsuitable for people on a weight-reducing diet.

109   Where or how do I find out about the carbohydrate or calorie content of food?

The BDA produce a booklet called *Countdown* which lists the carbohydrate and calorie content of most manufactured foods. It is divided into sections: green for foods which can be used regularly in the diet; amber for foods which can be used with a little more care; pink for foods which should only be used on special occasions. There is also detailed information on alcoholic drinks. Most bookshops sell small booklets called 'calorie counters' which list calorie values of many foods which can be carried in the pocket or handbag. Their greatest disadvantage is that the calories are calculated by the weight of the food and if you are away from home it is often difficult to know how much the particular food weighs.

110   I have just started tablets for my diabetes. Does this mean I can relax my diet?

No. Tablets are usually prescribed if diet alone is insufficient and the blood glucose level is not coming down to normal. If you start on tablets and relax your diet you are very likely to put on weight, and the blood glucose levels may climb even higher. The tablets must always be taken in conjunction with the diet advised by the dietitian.

*111   I have many family celebrations in the summer and
       would like advice on the choice of drinks. I have
       managed to lose weight and my control has improved
       so much that I have been taken off my diabetic tablets*

Any spirits are sugar free so could be a useful choice when
suitable sugar-free mixers or soda water are used with them.
Most red wines have a low sugar content and a couple of
glasses should not cause any problem. Some dry white wines
are also suitable such as Muscadet, white Macon or
Burgundy, dry Champagne, Soave, etc. Dry Vermouth can
also be drunk in small quantities. Diabetics who are weight
reducing would only be allowed very small quantities of
alcohol which would need to be counted as part of their diet
because of the calorie value of alcohol.

*112   Can I drink 'diet lagers' as part of my weight-reducing
       diet?*

'Low sugar' lagers such as Pils lager contain more alcohol
and calories than normal lagers and beers because they are
fermented longer to reduce the carbohydrate content.
Because of their high calorie content they are unsuitable for
diabetics trying to lose weight. Hemeling lager which
contains 75 Calories in a 275 ml can or Barbican alcohol-free
lager which contains 45 Calories in the same size can may be
more suitable for 'counting' in a weight-reducing diet.

113   Which scales do you recommend for weighing food?

It is not really necessary for diabetics to weigh their food. A
reasonable degree of accuracy is required to enable diabetics
to follow their diet properly but household measures are
quite accurate enough.

*114   I have a number of queries about my diet. Can you
       advise me how I can get advice about my diet?*

Good dietary advice is essential in the proper care of
diabetics and it needs to be tailored to fit every individual
diabetic. Most hospitals have a professional dietitian
attached to the diabetic clinic and some nurses and health

visitors who are specially trained in diabetes may also be able to give good dietary advice. Some general practitioners who organize their own diabetic clinic may arrange for a dietitian to visit this clinic. The BDA also offers helpful literature and advice but every diabetic should receive personal advice from a properly trained person.

115 Can you recommend any diabetic cookery books?

The BDA publish two very good cookery books called *Better Cookery for Diabetics* and *Cooking the New Diabetic Way* compiled by Jill Metcalfe. Another excellent cookery book is *The Diabetics' Diet Book* by Dr Jim Mann (published by Martin Dunitz). These books encourage the use of food that is higher in fibre and lower in fat. Diabetics on weight-reducing diets should note that some of the recipes are not necessarily low in calories and should take this into account when cooking from these books. A very recent publication which is to be highly recommended is *The Diabetics' Cookbook* written by Roberta Longstaff, SRD, and Dr Jim Mann and published by Martin Dunitz. This is a clear, well-illustrated book designed for family cooking as well as entertaining.

116 What is meant by the 'New Diet' for diabetics?

There are now new dietary recommendations for diabetics. The diabetic cannot cope with rapidly absorbed carbo-hydrate such as sweets or sugary foods, and therefore high-fibre carbohydrate foods which are absorbed slowly are more suited to the diabetic. Dietary fibre is of two main types: 'fibrous' fibres typically found in wholegrain cereals, wholemeal flour or bran, and 'viscous' fibres found in pulses (peas, beans and lentils) and some fruits and vegetables. Viscous fibres (especially those found in beans) appear to be of particular benefit to the diabetic because they slow down food absorption and hence the rate at which carbohydrate present in a meal will be absorbed into the bloodstream. All plant foods, especially those which are raw or only lightly cooked, are digested very slowly because of the plant-cell walls which have to be broken down before the carbohydrate contained within them is released.

The new recommendations are summed up as follows:

1. Excessive energy content (i.e. calories) in the diet worsens diabetic control. Therefore each patient requires a diet which does not contain a surplus amount of food energy and must be based on individual needs.

2. To lessen the risk of coronary heart disease and arterial disease the proportion of fat in the diet should be reduced. This may mean substituting skimmed milk for whole milk, using low-fat spreads instead of butter or margarine, greatly reducing the intake of cream and cheese and grilling rather than frying food, etc.

3. If the fat intake is reduced, the amount of carbohydrate can be increased to meet the energy needs of the diabetic. However, sugar and sugary foods must still be avoided and the carbohydrate should be slowly absorbed food, rich in fibre. This means eating more fruit, vegetables and beans, wholemeal bread instead of white, high-fibre cereals such as Weetabix, Shredded Wheat or All-bran, using wholemeal flour in baking, substituting brown rice for white rice and wholemeal pasta for ordinary pasta.

4. The diabetic who needs to lose weight no longer needs to follow a diet low in carbohydrate. The high-carbohydrate, low-fat diet is particularly suitable because it is a bulky diet and hence less likely to cause hunger.

5. Special diabetic foods are not encouraged because they are expensive and are usually high in calories. Low-calorie foods and drinks can be useful for those diabetics who need to lose weight.

6. Diabetics may have moderate amounts of alcohol provided its energy contribution is taken into account. Beers and lagers specially brewed for diabetics have a high alcohol and energy content and are not recommended.

117 When I was diagnosed diabetic last year I was told to lose 3 stone. Although it was difficult, I have managed to lose the weight and I am now down to my correct weight of 9 stone. However, I am very disappointed

*that I am still diabetic, and my urine tests still show
sugar. I thought the diabetes would disappear with the
fat.*

It is excellent that you have managed to lose the weight and
you must surely feel better and look better. It is sad that
your diabetes has not disappeared. Often reducing the
demand for insulin by reducing carbohydrate intake and by
losing weight means that a limited supply of natural insulin
is sufficient to balance the carbohydrate intake. Sometimes,
as has been true in your case, the deficiency of insulin is so
great that the diabetes persists, despite satisfactory weight
control. When this happens additional treatment with
tablets or even insulin may be required.

118 *My sister is a newly diagnosed diabetic who is having
to cope with a weight-reducing diet and giving up
smoking. Are there any sugar-free sweets she could
suck that will not upset her weight?*

We would suggest Trident or Orbit sugar-free chewing gum.
Both of these contain no sugar and the few calories per stick
should not upset her diet. Sugarless gums and sweets such
as those by Jacksons, Skels and Boots are also suitable. The
calorie values vary between 2 and 6 Cal per sweet so this
would need to be considered if many are eaten.

119 *I understand that all diabetics are being advised to use
less cheese but surely some cheeses contain less fat
than others. I have heard that Edam has little fat —
can I use more of this cheese?*

Edam does contain slightly less fat than cheeses such as
cheddar, but it is by no means a low-fat cheese when
compared with cottage cheese. There are other makes of
cheese, such as Tendale or St Ivel Shape cheese, which
contain less fat than those made in the traditional way — but
do not expect them to taste the same as their traditional
counterpart.

*120   I have not eaten carrots or parsnips for 10 years since I
       was diagnosed diabetic. A friend of mine has just
       developed diabetes and says she can eat them. Who is
       right?*

In the past few years dietitians and doctors have seen that
many vegetables contain some carbohydrate when analysed
in the laboratory but when they are eaten, the effect of the
carbohydrate is very small. Many clinics now tell diabetics
that they can eat most vegetables (except potatoes) in
moderate amounts without counting their carbohydrate
value.

Diet for diabetics on insulin (IDDM)

*121   Why do thin people taking insulin injections need a
       'diet'?*

The word 'diet' is often misleading as many people think of a
diet as being a weight-reducing diet. In fact the word diet
means a way of feeding or a prescribed course of food, and
for a diabetic simply means planned eating. The reason for
planning meals is to balance the amount of food against the
amount of insulin and exercise taken. When you take insulin
you need to consider the amount of carbohydrate eaten
throughout the day. Carbohydrate foods are starchy or
sugary foods such as bread, biscuits, potatoes, rice, fruit, ice
cream, etc. Proteins are an essential part of everyone's food
intake and are not restricted (unless you are overweight).
Examples of protein foods are meat, fish and eggs. Fats are
used for energy and are a more concentrated source of
calories than either carbohydrate or protein. Fats should
only be eaten in moderation as excess fat in the diet can lead
to being overweight or may contribute to heart disease in
later life. Examples of fats are butter, cream, margarine,
cheese (also a protein) and cooking oil.

Most people eat roughly the same amount of food each day
so when trying to balance food, insulin and exercise it makes
sense to keep the carbohydrate intake fairly constant so that
only the insulin or exercise needs to be adjusted. The aim of

the diet is to eat roughly the same amount of carbohydrate every day at much the same time each day. When you are first seen by the dietitian she will try to plan your diet so that there is not too much alteration from your previous eating pattern.

122 Why do diabetics taking insulin need to eat snacks in between meals?

When the pancreas functions normally, insulin is produced in response to eating food and 'switches off' when the food has been used up. With injected insulin this does not 'switch off' when no food has been eaten. As this insulin has a peak effect at certain times of the day it is important to cover the action of the insulin with a certain amount of carbohydrate otherwise a 'hypo' will occur. If you find it difficult to eat snacks in between meals it *may* be possible by changing from a short-acting insulin to an intermediate-acting insulin to cut down the number of snacks but most diabetics still need to eat snacks even when taking a longer acting insulin.

123 What are meant by 'exchanges'?

These are amounts of carbohydrate food measured in 10 grams (10 g) portions. 1 exchange = 10 g carbohydrate. Carbohydrate exchange lists can be very useful to add variety to your diet. A very comprehensive list is found in *Countdown* available from the BDA. Until you are used to the quantities of carbohydrate it is often helpful to weigh the food to begin with until you can judge the amount by eye and dispense with the weighing scales.

124 I have just started on insulin after many years of diet and tablets. How will my diet change?

If you need to reduce weight and have been on a weight-reducing diet it is unlikely that your diet will change very much but as a diabetic on insulin you will have to distribute the carbohydrate regularly through the day in order to avoid hypoglycaemia. If you are underweight or of normal weight the dietitian may recommend an increased carbohydrate intake.

125 As a diabetic taking insulin should I eat a bedtime snack?

Generally speaking, yes. As blood glucose tends to fall during the night it is sensible to cover the injected insulin with a snack before bed. Something like a milky drink with a couple of crispbreads or a slice of wholemeal bread would be suitable as it is carbohydrate that is fairly slowly absorbed and is more likely to last longer than for example a couple of semi-sweet biscuits.

126 My son has been putting on weight since being diagnosed diabetic 3 months ago. What are the reasons for this?

Most people lose weight before their diabetes is discovered and treated. This is because body fat is broken down for 'fuel' as glucose cannot be used properly. Also many calories are lost in the urine as sugar when the diabetes is uncontrolled. As soon as the control improves, the calories are retained, body fat is no longer broken down and the weight increases. If insulin-treated diabetics gain an excessive amount of weight this may be due to eating extra sugar and other carbohydrate to treat frequent hypo-glycaemia. In this case the dose of insulin should be reduced.

127 My 18-year-old daughter is diabetic and is trying to lose weight. She has an 80 gram carbohydrate diet and sticks to this rigidly. I cannot understand why she does not lose any weight

Just reducing the amount of carbohydrate eaten will not necessarily result in weight loss. When trying to lose weight it is important to reduce total calories which will involve also reducing protein and fat — particularly fat as it is a concentrated form of calories. Your daughter should avoid fried foods, sugary foods and alcohol, cut down her cheese intake, substitute skimmed milk for ordinary milk and allow only a scraping of butter or margarine on her bread. A diet that is higher in fibre will be more satisfying and encourage greater weight loss than a very low fibre, low-carbohydrate diet. It is important to avoid hypoglycaemia as constantly treating hypos will result in a weight gain and it is probable that the dose of insulin will need to be reduced.

128 *I am an insulin-dependent diabetic. Why am I told not to eat sugar in my diet and yet have to carry sugar in my pocket?*

Sugar or foods containing large amounts of sugar are absorbed into the bloodstream very quickly. Insulin injections do not work that quickly and cannot cope with this sudden surge in blood glucose, which leads to poor diabetic control. However, this sudden rise in blood glucose can be useful if the blood glucose level is low and you are feeling hypo because you will need something that is absorbed very quickly. This is why you should always carry sugar, glucose or sweets in your pocket so you can treat a hypo immediately.

129 *What is the best thing to take when I have a hypo?*

Some form of rapidly absorbed carbohydrate is ideal. This can be neat sugar as sugar lumps, or sugar in sweets (not diabetic sweets). If you are at home Lucozade is excellent and small beakers can be obtained from the BDA which measure the Lucozade in 10 g portions. The best thing to carry in your pocket are glucose tablets such as Dextrosol as they are absorbed very quickly. They are also less likely to be eaten when not hypo than ordinary sweets! We would not recommend carrying chocolate in your pocket as the temptation to eat it may be great, and if it is not eaten it makes a mess!

130 *What are the best sugar substitutes to use?*

The three main sugar substitutes are fructose, sorbitol, and saccharin. Fructose is a carbohydrate which occurs naturally in many fruits and does not require insulin for its metabolism. It is about one-and-a-half times as sweet as table sugar but contains as many calories as ordinary sugar and is not therefore suitable for the overweight. It can be used in cooking very satisfactorily but the BDA recommend that no more than 50 g (weight) is consumed in any one day.

Sorbitol is a sweetening agent which has no significant effect upon the blood sugar level. It is about half as sweet as table sugar but has the same number of calories as sugar so should not be used by those who need to lose weight. It is useful in baking and has some preservative qualities so is widely used in the making of diabetic jam. Its greatest disadvantage is that eating large quantities will produce wind and diarrhoea and its use should therefore be limited to no more than 50 g (weight) per day.

Saccharin is a synthetic sweetener which has over 500 times the sweetening power of table sugar and is calorie free so is very suitable for people on a weight-reducing diet. It is inclined to have a bitter after-taste which is more prominent if it has been heated. Where possible saccharine should be added to food after it has been cooked. It is available in tablet or liquid form.

Cyclamate sweeteners are also synthetic sweeteners. Although they are available in some countries they have been banned in the UK and the USA as some doubts were cast on their safety. They have a less bitter after-taste when used in cooking. Powdered artificial sweeteners are best avoided as some contain sugar, e.g. Sweet n'low, Sweetex powder, Sucron.

131　What are the new 'intense' sweeteners?

They are called aspartame, acesulfane-K and thaumatin. Saccharin is also an 'intense' sweetener but has been in use for 100 years.

Aspartame, also known by its trade name Nutra Sweet, is a low-calorie sweetener made from two synthetically produced amino acids, L-aspartic acid and L-phenylalanine. It is 200 times sweeter than sucrose. The manufacturers claim that it tastes very like sugar without the bitterness associated with saccharin. Sold under the brand name Canderel, it comes in either tablets or sachets of powder combined with a bulking agent. It is, however, much more expensive than saccharin. It loses its sweetness at high temperatures and should be added to food after cooking.

Drinks containing aspartame now on the market are — Diet Coke, Diet Pepsi, Diet Rola Cola, Diet Spring-Up, Energen One Cal, Orangina, Diet Quosh, Diet Corona, Diet Tango and Schweppes Slimline Drinks.

Acesulfane-K is a low-calorie sweetener made from an organic salt. It is 200 times sweeter than sugar. It is available in the shops in tablet form as Hermesetas Gold or Sweetex Plus and although it costs more than saccharin, is less expensive then aspartame.

Thaumatin, trade name Talin, is the third new intense sweetener. It is a naturally occurring protein extracted from the West African Katemfe fruit, and at 2000–3000 times the sweetness of sugar it is the sweetest substance known to man. The perception of the sweet taste is delayed and it will probably be used as a flavour extender in pharmaceutical products, e.g. toothpaste, or used in combination with other sweeteners in soft drinks. It is unlikely to be sold on its own as a table-top sweetener.

None of the 'intense' sweeteners can be used successfully in recipes where sugar provides bulk, e.g. cakes and biscuits, or where sugar acts as a preservative, e.g. jam.

132 Are low-calorie foods and drinks suitable for diabetics?

Many tinned fruits are now sold with no sweetener added and would therefore be suitable if the calorie and carbo-hydrate content is counted in the day's allowance. Some jams and marmalades are also sold without sweetening agents but because they do not contain added sugar do not keep well once opened. Low-calorie soups and 'instant meals' may be used providing the carbohydrate and calorie content is taken into consideration. These should be printed on the label. If they are not, do not use them.

Low-calorie fruit squash available in supermarkets should not be used as it may contain sugar, but Boots low-calorie squash is fine. Any of the drinks listed can be taken in unlimited quantities. Fresca, Energen One-Cal, Diet Pepsi, Roses and Boots diabetic cordials, PLJ, Schweppes slimline drinks, Hunts, Club and Canada Dry low-calorie drinks, Weight-Watchers drinks, Diet Spring-up, Orangina, Diet Quosh, Diet Corona, Diet Tango.

133   Why do diabetic foods cost so much?

The market for diabetic foods is much smaller and as a result production costs are higher. In addition sorbitol is commonly used as a sweetening agent which is more expensive than sugar.

134   My daughter has been diabetic for 4 years and has had no problems with her diet. She takes part in most school sports but since she has taken up running longer distances she finds that she has a hypo about 2 hours after she has finished running. She has no problems during the run so what should she eat to counteract this?

The effect of exercise on the body can last well after the exercise has stopped. The muscles are restocking their energy stores (glycogen). Any food taken lasts during the exercise but runs out later on. She will benefit from taking an extra carbohydrate snack (such as a sandwich or two) after the run has finished.

135   Why is it on a carbohydrate-controlled diet I have to 'count' milk but can eat cheese freely?

Milk contains some carbohydrate in the form of milk sugar and has to be included in your carbohydrate-controlled diet. Cheese is made from the fatty portion of milk and during the making the carbohydrate is left behind in the whey. Full-fat cheeses are almost carbohydrate free but because they are high-calorie, high-fat foods, they should only be used in small amounts.

136   My son is getting a diabetic Easter egg this Easter but I am a little anxious about the amount of sorbitol in it

Most Easter eggs contain 30–40 g sorbitol. If this was eaten all at once it might cause a stomach upset so it would be sensible to eat small amounts to last over the whole of the Easter holiday.

137 Should I increase my insulin over Christmas to cope with the extra food I will be eating?

Certainly extra insulin can be taken to cover extra carbohydrate that may be eaten at Christmas and on special occasions. You will probably work out by trial and error how much the insulin needs to be adjusted but to begin with we would suggest that you do not increase the insulin by more than 4 units at a time. Remember that if you do this too often you will be very likely to put on too much weight!

138 I have been following Lawrence Lines for many years but have recently been told that the Dr Lawrence diet is old fashioned. What is used instead?

Although Lawrence Lines are not used these days the system is not so very different from our present diet exchanges. These days carbohydrate is calculated in 10 g portions which is roughly equivalent to 1 black Lawrence line. The red lines which are protein and fat are largely ignored.

139 My doctor has suggested that I take guar gum before my meals in an attempt to improve my blood glucose levels. What is guar gum and how can it improve my control?

Guar gum has been shown to lower the blood glucose levels after a meal in both diabetic and non-diabetic subjects and, as a result, may improve diabetic control in some patients. Guar gum is derived from the cluster bean and is a high source of dietary fibre. It works by forming a viscous gel in the gut which results in a delayed absorption of carbohydrate. Until recently, its main drawback has been its unpalatability but there are now new palatable sources of guar gum, manufactured under the names of Lejguar (Britannia Pharmaceuticals Ltd), Guarem granules (Rybar Laboratories Ltd) and Glucotard (M C P Pharmaceuticals Ltd). Both Lejguar and Guarem granules can be mixed with water or fruit juice, and are taken before or during a meal and are quite tasteless. Glucotard comes in the form of lemon-flavoured, large granules which are placed dry on the tongue and swallowed with several mouthfuls of water. Because guar keeps the stomach fuller for longer, it can reduce the appetite in people who need to lose weight. The disadvantages of using it are increased wind, and it may have a laxative effect initially.

Overweight (obesity)

140 I have just been told that I have diabetes. Is it true that if I lose weight I will probably not need insulin injections?

Most people with diabetes in the UK do not need insulin — especially those over 40 years old who are overweight. People who are a normal weight at the time of diagnosis are more likely to need insulin or tablets. In overweight diabetics, it is impossible to predict how much weight a particular patient will need to lose in order to control the diabetes. Sometimes the loss of half a stone (3 kg) is enough to restore the blood glucose to normal while other patients remain diabetic after losing several stones by dieting. Such people may then need tablets or even insulin, but provided they do not become *too* thin, they will be better off for shedding the excess weight.

141 I have been diabetic on insulin for 8 years and over this time I have put on a lot of weight. My doctor says that insulin does not make you fat, but if that is so why have I put on so much weight?

People tend to lose weight if their diabetes is badly controlled. This is mainly because they are losing a lot of sugar which is equivalent to calories in their urine. Once the diabetes is controlled sugar is no longer lost in the urine and so there will be a tendency for a diabetic starting treatment to put on weight. Insulin in the right dose does not make people fat but anyone having too much insulin will have to eat more to prevent hypos and these extra calories will cause an increase in weight. If a diabetic on insulin does become too fat, losing the extra weight can be a slow business. People taking insulin cannot afford the luxury of sudden, drastic dieting but can only lose weight by careful reduction of both food and insulin. This can be a delicate balance but many diabetics manage it successfully.

It is best not to put on weight in the first place and there is a particular risk of this at the time when children stop growing. Children need enormous amounts of food when they are actually growing taller but once fully grown a conscious effort must be made to reduce the total food intake. Girls usually stop growing a year or two after their first period and unless they eat a lot less at that stage they will almost certainly become fat — and it is much easier to put on weight than to take it off.

142   I have heard that tablets for diabetics can make you fat. Is this true?

Tablets can only make you overweight if used wrongly. Sulphonylureas (e.g. chlorpropamide and glibenclamide) work by making the failing pancreas produce more insulin. An overweight diabetic who is not in urgent need of insulin should first of all get down to his or her normal weight and then take tablets if the blood glucose is still raised. If an overweight diabetic is started on tablets straightaway without first trying the effect of diet, that person will find it difficult to lose weight and may become even fatter. In other words tablets should not be used as a substitute for diet and weight reduction.

Unproved methods of treatment

143   Is vitamin E beneficial to diabetics?

Vitamins are substances needed in very small quantities in the diet to prevent certain diseases. Thus minute amounts of vitamin D are needed for the manufacture of normal bone, but vitamin D taken in large quantities may actually cause serious illness.

Vitamin E does not seem to be needed at all by humans and people deprived of it do not come to any harm. In rats it is a different story, for if they are fed on a diet containing no vitamin E their sexual organs stop working. However, vitamin E causes no benefit to humans — not even to diabetics.

144 *Daily doses of Sanatogen tonic wine have helped the neuropathy in my legs and I wonder if Sanatogen treatment will eventually lead to a complete cure of the muscular pains and weakness? Is there any other treatment known to be successful?*

Sanatogen is not a recommended treatment for painful legs though the small amounts of alcohol it contains may help to relieve the pain. The pain from neuropathy may come and go at different times but it is hard to see how a tonic wine could cause any permanent improvement. The only hope in cases of painful neuropathy is to control the blood glucose extremely carefully.

145 *Recently I saw a physical training expert demonstrating the technique of achieving complete relaxation. She concluded by saying, 'Of course, this is not suitable for everyone, for example diabetics.' Is this true and, if so, why?*

This sounds like an example of ignorant discrimination against diabetics. There is no reason why diabetics should not practise complete relaxation if they want to. If the session went on for a long time you might have to miss a snack or even a meal but as you are burning up so little energy in a relaxed state, perhaps that would not matter.

146 *My back has troubled me for many years and a friend has suggested that as a last resort I should try acupuncture. Would there be any objection to this, given that I am a diabetic? Might it even help my diabetes?*

Acupuncture has been a standard form of medical treatment in China for 5000 years. In the last 20 years it has become more widely used in this country. In China acupuncture has always been thought of as a way of preventing disease and is less effective in treating illness. In the UK acupuncture tends to be the last resort of people who have been ill (and usually in pain) for a long time. It is most often tried in such conditions as a painful back, where orthodox medicine often fails to help. Most doctors in this country feel that acupuncture is unlikely to help a bad back but it is worth a try if all else has failed — at least it will not do any harm. Even practitioners of the art do not claim that acupuncture can cure diabetes.

147 I have heard that there are herbal remedies for diabetes. Could you enlarge on these?

There have been many plants which are said to reduce the high level of blood glucose in diabetics. One of these is a berry from West Africa and another a tropical plant called Karela, or Bitter Gourd. These only have a mild effect on lowering the blood glucose and as the Bitter Gourd lives up to its name and tastes disgusting, you would find conventional tablets more convenient, more reliable and much safer. Herbal remedies have no effect on diabetics who need insulin.

148 My little girl has just contracted diabetes at the age of three. I would do anything to cure her. Would hypnosis be worth a try?

Most parents have this desperate desire for a cure when their child becomes diabetic. In one sense, then, insulin injections are a cure in that they replace the missing hormone. This fact is not much consolation to the parent. Although this sense of desperation is a natural reaction, it is best for your child's sake to try to accept that she is likely to remain diabetic. In this way she is more likely to come to terms with the condition herself. It is natural to grieve for a time but then you must face facts as a family and make use of all the help that is available for you and your daughter. In that way she will be less upset about her diabetes than you are. Hypnosis will not help her insulin cells to regenerate.

149 *An evangelistic healing crusade claims to heal among other diseases 'sugar diabetes', malignant growth and multiple sclerosis, etc. Are these claims correct?*

There are of course a handful of reports of miracle cures of various serious diseases like cancer but these are few and far between. A mild overweight diabetic might be persuaded to lose weight by a faith healer and it might appear that his diabetes was 'cured' but no diabetic on insulin has benefited from a healing crusade except in the strictly spiritual sense.

150 *I recently read an article on ginseng which said it was beneficial to diabetics. Have you any information on this?*

Ginseng comes from Korea and the powdered root is said to have amazing properties. You may come across glossy leaflets extolling the virtues of ginseng and implying that it will cure all conceivable ailments, as well as increasing your sexual prowess. The cost of these lavish booklets is passed on to any customer gullible enough to buy them. Ginseng does not help diabetics — or anyone else for that matter.

3

Monitoring and control

Introduction

The key to a successful life with diabetes is achieving good blood glucose control. The degree of success can be judged only by measurements of the body's response to treatment. Unfortunately, the mere fact that a diabetic feels well does *not* mean that he or she is well controlled. It is only when control goes *badly* wrong that the person is aware that something is amiss and by then it may be too late; if the blood glucose is too low the diabetic may be aware of 'hypo' symptoms and if untreated may progress to unconsciousness ('hypoglycaemic coma'). At the other end of the spectrum, when the blood glucose concentration rises very steeply, the diabetic will be aware initially of increased thirst and urination, and if untreated this may progress to nausea, vomiting, weakness and eventual clouding of consciousness (and coma). It has long been apparent that relying on how one feels is too imprecise, even though some people may be able to 'feel' subtle changes in their control. For this reason, there have been developed many different tests to allow precise measurement of the goodness (or badness) of control and as the years go by, these tests get better and better. The involvement of the patient in monitoring and control of their own condition has always been essential for successful treatment. With the development of the more modern methods (such as blood glucose monitoring), this has become even more apparent; it allows the diabetic to measure precisely how effective they are at balancing the conflicting forces of diet, exercise and insulin, and to make adjustments in order to maintain this balance.

In the early days after the discovery of insulin, urine tests were the only tests available and it required a small laboratory even to do these. It was necessary for the patient to boil a sample of urine in a test tube with Benedict's reagent. This test was simplified considerably by the Ames Company when they introduced Clinitest tablets. These are still widely used though many people find dipsticks (e.g. Diastix or Diabur 5000) more convenient.

Urine tests have always had the disadvantage that they are only an indirect indicator of what the diabetic really needs to know — that is the concentration (level) of glucose in the blood. Blood glucose monitoring first became available to patients in 1977 and since then has become widely accepted. Despite the disadvantage of having to prick a finger to get a drop of blood, the increased accuracy and directness of this test has been much appreciated. Blood glucose monitoring allows a fine balance between diet, insulin and exercise to be maintained and, as far as one can see, will remain the most important monitoring procedure for the future.

As anyone who has monitored glucose concentrations in the blood will know, these vary considerably throughout the day as well as from day to day. For this reason, a single reading at a twice yearly visit to the local diabetic clinic is of limited value in assessing long-term success or failure with control. The recent introduction of haemoglobin A_{1c} (glycosylated haemoglobin or HbA_1) measurements (p.129) has given the patients and doctors a very reliable test for longer term monitoring of the average blood glucose level (taking into account the moment to moment peaks and troughs) over an interval of 2–3 months before the test was done. Attainment of a normal HbA_1 level indicates that the blood glucose concentration has been contained within the limits of normal and indicates to patient and doctor alike that providing there are not unacceptable attacks of hypoglycaemia, balance is excellent and no further manipulation is required. It can readily be seen that attaining a normal HbA$_1$ and maintaining it at normal is an important goal for patient and doctor. Not all can achieve it, but it is within the reach of most patients and having once got there, it is most important to strive to maintain a normal HbA$_1$, since this is undoubtedly the most effective way of eliminating the risk of long-term diabetic 'complications'.

Monitoring of other aspects of health are an important part of long-term diabetic care. Regular checks on eyes, blood pressure and feet are a good way of picking up conditions that require treatment at a stage before they have done any serious damage.

Control and monitoring

1 *I am an 18-year-old diabetic on insulin. When my sugar is high I do not feel any ill effects. Is it really necessary for me to maintain strict control?*

It is quite true that some diabetics do not develop the typical thirst or dry mouth, frequency of passing water or tiredness which usually occur if the blood glucose is high and diabetes out of control. Of course it is much more difficult for a diabetic in this situation — such as yourself — to sense when control is poor and take steps to improve it. Yet if you lack these symptoms, blood glucose control is still important because the development of 'complications' after many years is much less likely and possibly even eliminated if you can maintain blood glucose concentrations within the normal range. You will clearly depend on your blood tests to determine your control.

2 *We are told that good blood glucose control will avoid complications in the future. What is the nature of these threatened complications and how long do they take to occur?*

Complications are dealt with in detail in Chapter 8 but here it is important to say that as far as we can see all the long-term complications of diabetes are most common in those with poor blood glucose control and are almost certainly a consequence of having a blood glucose level which is higher than normal. Experimental evidence indicates very strongly that if you keep your blood glucose level in the normal range you avoid exposing yourself to these risks. These complications take a long time to develop but once they have occurred they are very difficult to reverse.

3 *In the past 12 months I have had to increase my insulin dosage several times yet I was still unable to get a urine test below 2%. I have been diabetic for 25 years and until last year I have always been well controlled. Can you advise me what to do?*

There are many reasons why diabetic control might gradually deteriorate and increased insulin be needed after many years of good control. These include:

a   Any change in your way of life leading to a decrease in physical activity such as normally occurs as we all get older.
b   Some slight alteration in dietary habits.
c   Almost any illness including chronic infections, and also stress, emotional upsets and depression.
d   Some technical problem relating to insulin injections such as the repeated use of one site so the absorption of insulin becomes less regular and complete.
e   Increase in weight and a tendency to middle-age spread (this can be reversed by appropriate dieting and weight loss).
f   Finally there are more subtle variations in insulin requirements from time to time due to alterations within the body's metabolism which in the non-diabetic go undetected as the pancreas automatically compensates. The diabetic has to increase (or decrease) the total insulin dosage to maintain balance.

4 *Can stress influence blood glucose readings?*

Yes, but the response varies from one person to another. In some people stress tends to make the blood glucose rise whereas in other people it may increase the risk of hypoglycaemia.

5 *Would I be able to achieve better control if I went on to three injections a day?*

The exact methods of obtaining good control in diabetes varies considerably from one person to another. In some mild cases good control can be achieved by dietary means alone: the more severe cases need tablets, whereas in the most severe cases the blood glucose can only be brought under control with insulin injections. Amongst the patients who are treated with insulin some can be well controlled on one injection a day, the majority require two injections a day and in some good control can only be achieved by three or more injections a day or more recently by the use of insulin pumps. The body normally produces insulin in response to every meal and for this reason one might expect that good control could only be achieved with multiple injections of insulin to cover every meal. In practice this is seldom necessary but should be considered if you cannot obtain normal blood glucose and HbA_1 on your current regimen.

Blood glucose

6 *What is the normal range of blood glucose in a non-diabetic?*

Before meals the range is from 3.5 to 5.5 mmol/l. After meals it may rise as high as 7–10 mmol/l depending on the carbohydrate content of the meal. However long a non-diabetic person goes without food the blood glucose concentration never drops below 3 mmol/l and however much they eat it never goes above 10 mmol/l.

7 *My blood glucose monitor is calculated in millimoles. Can you tell me what a millimole is?*

Formerly blood glucose was measured in milligrams per 100 millilitres (mg%; mg per dl) of blood. To conform with a

Système Internationale adopted by the Common Market the unit was changed to millimoles per litre (mmol/l of blood). The conversion is as follows:

1 mmol/l = 18 mg%
2 mmol/l = 36 mg%
3 mmol/l = 54 mg%
4 mmol/l = 72 mg%
5 mmol/l = 90 mg%
6 mmol/l = 108 mg%
7 mmol/l = 126 mg%
8 mmol/l = 144 mg%
9 mmol/l = 162 mg%
10 mmol/l = 180 mg%
12 mmol/l = 216 mg%
15 mmol/l = 270 mg%
20 mmol/l = 360 mg%
22 mmol/l = 396 mg%
25 mmol/l = 459 mg%
30 mmol/l = 540 mg%.

8 Are the new blood glucose meters suitable for tablet-controlled diabetics?

All diabetics whether controlled by diet, tablets or insulin should strive for perfect control. Traditionally this has been achieved by regular urine tests at home. Since 1977 there has been a move towards encouraging patients to do their own blood glucose measurements. This form of monitoring was thought to be most suitable for insulin-treated patients. However, further experience has shown that it is equally suited to tablet and diet-treated patients. The disadvantage of having to prick one's finger to obtain a drop of blood is more than compensated for by the increased accuracy and reliability of the readings so obtained.

9 Should I keep my sticks for blood glucose monitoring in the fridge with my insulin?

No. It is important to keep them dry as any moisture will impair their activity. You must put the lid back on the container immediately after removing a strip. The strips contain enzymes which are biological substances which do not last forever. Once a bottle of sticks is opened, write the date of opening on the bottle and use its contents within the recommended period (BM Test Glycemie 20-800 R, 6 months; Dextrostix, 4 months; Visidex II, 6 months; foil-wrapped sticks may be used until the expiry date stamped on each foil — up to 2 years). Although the sticks should not be kept in the refrigerator it is important that they are not exposed to extremely high temperatures and should be kept in cool, well-shaded areas. The life of a bottle of sticks is very much reduced in hot weather, and you must not leave them in hot places such as the glove box or boot of a car. If the sticks have gone off they may look normal before use, but will tend to give a falsely low reading; Dextrostix and Visidex II are provided with zero colour blocks. Before use check that the sticks match the blocks to ensure they are in good condition. If you ever have reason to suspect the result of a blood test the best thing is to repeat the test using a new bottle of sticks.

10 How are the enzymes on the test strip made?

Enzymes are biological substances extracted from living cells, sometimes plants, sometimes animals, sometimes bacteria. The enzymes on the test strips are a mixture obtained from plants.

11 Why is it that equipment to aid diabetes is not all free of charge as it is a life-long condition and people with other life-long diseases are entitled to such benefits?

Most of the traditional equipment for diabetic control is available free on prescription. However, more recently as new techniques are developed the government has found it increasingly difficult to make these available without increasing the amount of money spent on health. It is also partly a failure of the organization of the National Health Service to keep pace with new developments. The best way that you can favourably influence this is by lobbying your Member of Parliament and asking him this question.

*12 I have read about home blood glucose monitoring and
would like to do this myself but my hospital clinic does
not supply the sticks as they say they are too expensive.
A friend of mine who attends another clinic can obtain
the sticks on prescription from her clinic. Why is there
such a difference between hospitals?*

As blood sugar reagent sticks are not available on the drug
tariff, i.e. on prescription from a general practitioner,
patients either have to buy the sticks themselves or they
may be obtained on prescription via a hospital pharmacy.
The major problem is that many hospitals are unable to
afford this expenditure and therefore will not supply them.
We think that all diabetic patients should have the
opportunity of monitoring blood glucose levels at home if
they wish. If you are unable to obtain sticks free of charge
then you should write to your Member of Parliament to
complain. Alternatively or additionally you can write to the
Health Service Ombudsman at Church House, Great Smith
Street, London SW1.

*13 I had a glucose tolerance test and my highest blood
sugar was 17 mmol/l. However my urine analysis was
negative for sugar. Is there a way I could test my blood
for sugar without going to the laboratory?*

You clearly have a 'high renal threshold' to glucose (p.126)
which means that it is only at very high concentrations of
sugar in the blood that any sugar escapes into the urine. In
your case urine tests are unhelpful and blood tests essential.

Self-monitoring of blood glucose by diabetic patients first
started in 1977 and has rapidly spread. There are many
different techniques, most of them based on reagent sticks
containing enzymes that react to the glucose in the blood and
produce a colour which is deeper as the concentration of
glucose in the blood rises. The three most widely used strips
at present are Dextrostix, Visidex II and BM Test Glycemie
20-800 R. Although the colour that develops on the strip can
be matched with a scale of colours on the container by eye, it
is possible to make this reading more effective with some
strips by use of a specially designed meter which gives a

direct reading of the glucose concentration in the blood in either mmol/l or mg/dl. Some people find that they can read the colour reaction adequately by eye alone but many patients prefer the objectivity of a meter. Unfortunately the meters cost anywhere between £50 and £120 and are not available on prescription. They should last for at least 5 years and most patients who have purchased these meters consider their investment worthwhile. The choice of which stick to use and whether to use a meter is an important one and should not be made without discussing the possibilities in detail with an expert. Most hospital diabetic clinics will now be able to show patients the various techniques that are available. The selection of which stick and which meter is best made by the patient after they have made a survey of what is available. All the different methods give good results provided they are used sensibly and after proper instruction (*see* Figures 3, 4 and 5).

14   When I am in a hypo I cannot read the colours on blood test sticks. What do you advise?

In your case it would clearly be preferable for you to have a meter that will read the colour of the sticks for you and give you a direct reading of your blood glucose. People vary in their ability to read the colours on Dextrostix, Visidex or BM Test Glycemie 20-800 R sticks. Some find it difficult, others find it easy. Even some of those who find it easy do not make very accurate measurements. If you read the sticks without using a meter you must sometimes check your accuracy against a laboratory method or somebody else's meter. You also draw attention in your question to the fact that when hypoglycaemic there may be a deterioration in vision and failure of concentration — both of which increase the chance of error.

Figure 3   Techniques for blood glucose testing using BM Test Glycemie 20-800 R or BM Test BG strips.

a. Wash and dry hands. Do not use spirit on skin. Prick side or pulp of finger or thumb with suitable lancet.

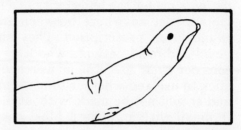

b. Squeeze *gently* until large drop forms.

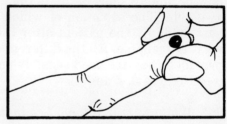

c. Gently turn hand until drop hangs from finger.

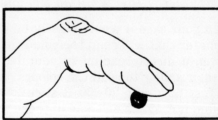

d. Touch blood on test pad. Do not spread or smear the blood.

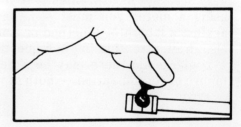

e. Leave blood on test pad for *one minute*. This pad should be covered completely with the blood standing 'proud' on the strip.

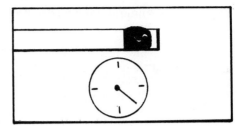

f. Hold strip against a flat surface and wipe blood away *gently* three times with a clean pad of cotton wool.

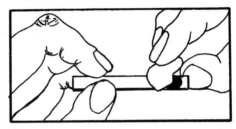

Leave test pad for one further minute and compare colour with label on tin or insert into meter.

When using *BM Test Glycemie 20-800 R* if the reading at 2 minutes is above 13 mmol/l, leave for a further minute and read again.

When reading values below 7 mmol/l give priority to the block which matches the lower blue test zone. For values above 7 mmol/l give priority to the block which matches the colour on the upper beige/green zone.

Record the result.

Figure 4   Technique for blood glucose testing using Dextrostix.

a. Wash and dry hands. Do not use spirit on skin. Prick side of finger or pulp of finger or thumb with suitable lancet.

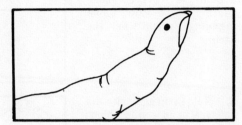

b. Squeeze *gently* until large drop forms.

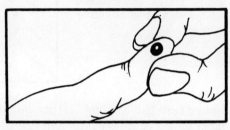

c. Turn hand until drop hangs from finger and apply blood freely to the entire reagent pad.

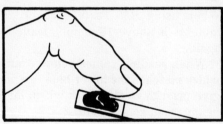

d. Time reaction for *exactly 60 seconds*. The test pad must be completely covered and remain shiny and moist with blood for the time of the reaction. If only a thin film is spread over the area, throw the stick away and start again.

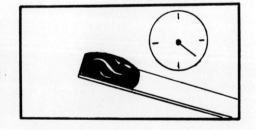

e. At one minute, immediately wash all the blood from the test strip with a sharp stream of water using a wash bottle directed just above the reagent area.

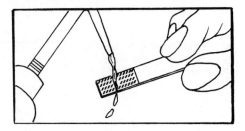

f. Blot the reagent pad of the strip on absorbent tissue. Insert immediately into the meter and take the reading.

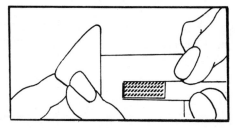

Record the result.

Figure 5 Technique for blood glucose testing using Visidex II.

a. Wash and dry hands. Do not use spirit on skin. Prick side or pulp of finger or thumb with suitable lancet.

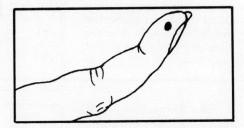

b. Squeeze *gently* until large drop forms.

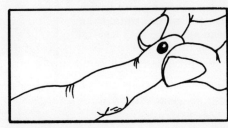

c. Turn hand until drop hangs from finger.

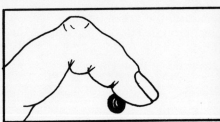

d. Apply blood freely to cover both reagent pads.

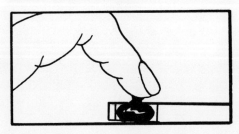

e. Leave the blood on the pads for *exactly 30 seconds*. The test pads must remain shiny and moist with blood for the time of the reaction.

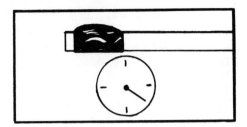

f. Remove the blood either by blotting the strip once on absorbent tissue or by wiping the pads *gently* once or twice with a cotton wool ball. Wait an *additional 90 seconds* (2 minutes from applying the blood) before comparing pads to the colour charts.

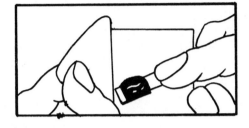

Compare the green pad to the nearest matching green colour block. If the green block is darker than the 6 mmol/l colour block compare the lower pad to the nearest matching orange colour block.

Record the result.

15   I feel hypo when my blood glucose is normal and only feel well when it is high. I feel very ill when my doctor tries to keep my blood glucose normal. Am I hooked on a high blood sugar?

You report a most interesting and potentially very dangerous state of affairs. In a diabetic patient with poor control for several years, the brain and the other tissues in the body can adjust themselves to a high concentration of glucose in the blood. As a result they may feel hypo at a time when their blood glucose is normal or even high. The long-term outlook for patients such as this is poor unless they can be re-educated to tolerate normal blood glucose levels without feeling unwell. This is possible but requires determination on behalf of the patient and an understanding of the long-term dangers of a high blood glucose. This problem can be overcome only if the patient is prepared to measure his own blood glucose level. He must accept that however unwell he feels no harm will be done if the blood glucose remains above 3 mmol/l.

16   Apart from the initial day or two after diagnosis I have had no glucose in my urine at any time since I have been on treatment with 100 gram carbohydrate diet and metformin. I feel lost without an occasional blood sugar for guidance, so can you suggest any guidelines for me?

If you check your urine 2 hours after a meal and the tests consistently remain negative for glucose, you need to ascertain what sort of levels the blood glucose reaches before you show any sugar in the urine. You can either do this by making a note of the results of the blood tests that you had when you went to the diabetic clinic or to your GP and relate those to urine tests or by learning how to do your own blood glucose readings and making a study yourself at home. Consistently negative urine tests used to be regarded as an indication of satisfactory diabetic control. We now know that this is not always the case and that some people can still have negative urine tests at a time when their blood glucose is quite high. Our criteria for good diabetic control at present is blood glucose readings within the range 3–10 mmol/l with an average of approximately 5 and a haemoglobin A_1 of less than 8.5%. If you can achieve this simply by monitoring your urine then that is all that is strictly necessary but it sounds as if you would feel happier if you gave up urine testing and adopted blood testing as your regular monitoring routine.

17 *Is there a way of knowing how much extra Actrapid insulin to give depending on my blood glucose level so I can maintain a better blood glucose?*

The answer is yes, but it will require some experimenting on your behalf. The particular type and dose of insulin most suited to you can be best judged by repeated measurements of your body's response to the insulin that you are taking. If you find, for example, that your blood glucose always goes very high after breakfast then you may be able to prevent this by taking more Actrapid before breakfast, but before making any adjustment in insulin dosage it is important to see that the blood glucose changes you see are part of a regular pattern. This is part of the process of balancing insulin, diet and exercise and we would caution against taking an extra dose of insulin if you come across a rather high blood glucose reading as an isolated finding. It is usually far better to try to work out a routine whereby you can prevent the blood glucose from rising too high rather than to take an extra injection of insulin when it has happened. There are exceptions to this rule of course. If you suddenly become unwell and your blood glucose goes very high, repeated extra injections of a short-acting insulin such as Actrapid is the most effective way of preventing the development of ketoacidosis (p.277).

18 *I find that my control is only good for one week and that is the week before my period. Why is this and what should I do about it?*

In some people the dose of insulin required to control diabetes varies in relation to the menstrual cycle. Your question implies that you become more sensitive to insulin in the week before you menstruate and you probably require more insulin at the other times in your cycle. There is no reason why you should not try to work out a pattern where you reduce the insulin dose the week before your period and increase it at other times. This variation is due to different hormones coming from the ovary during the menstrual cycle. Some of these hormones have an anti-insulin effect. The same sort of effects may occur when taking oral contraceptive tablets and whilst pregnant. The correct thing to do is to make adjustments in the insulin dose in order to compensate for these hormonal changes and to keep the balance of the blood glucose where it should be.

19 Where is the best place to obtain blood for measuring blood glucose levels?

It is usually easiest to obtain blood from the fingertips. You can use either the pulp which is the fleshy part of the fingertip, the sides of the fingertips or some people like to use the area just below the nail bed. Most people find it easier to use the tip but the sides of the fingertips are less sensitive than the pulp and it may be necessary for some people such as guitarists, pianists or typists to avoid the finger pulp.

The fleshy ear lobes are also suitable areas for obtaining blood and are less sensitive than the fingers but they can be difficult to use as the blood has to be applied to the reagent stick with the aid of a mirror. The ear lobes are a useful area for children if the parents are obtaining the blood for the child.

20 What is the best 'finger-pricker'?

We would recommend the use of Monolet (from Mariner Medical, Medistron Ltd or Hypoguard Ltd) or Unilet (from Owen Mumford Ltd) blood lancets either on their own or in conjunction with an automatic device (Plate 8). These lancets usually obtain a good drop of blood without leaving a painful wound. If these lancets are not available disposable needles such as are used for an insulin injection may be used. We would deter anyone from using the pressed steel pointed blades which are still commonly seen in hospitals. Although they obtain a good drop of blood they leave a painful wound which can take a long time to heal.

21 *I have trouble pricking my fingers with a blood lancet. What can you recommend?*

Firstly make sure that you are using good lancets such as Monolets or Unilets and not pressed steel lancets. If you have trouble pushing the lancet in quickly you may find an automatic device helpful. Two commonly used devices are the Autolet which fires the lancet quickly into the finger by pushing a button, or the Autoclix which encloses a Monolet in a spring-loaded case and prevents you from seeing the lancet prick the finger. The Autoclix comes with three different platforms for use with varying thickness of skin. A recent introduction to the market is the Monojecter which is designed to hold a Monolet lancet. Gentle pressure releases the spring-loaded lancet to a controlled depth and retracts it, keeping the lancet out of sight. Another helpful lancet is the Mini-Lancet which comes with its own outer case which controls the depth of penetration and enables the user to pierce the skin quickly. The Auto-Lancet has two different sized tips supplied — one for adult use and one for childrens' use. It is a spring-loaded device which hides the Monolet from view during operation (*see* Plate 8).

For a list of finger pricking devices, *see* p.116.

22 *Should I clean my fingers with spirit or antiseptic before pricking them?*

We do not recommend the use of spirit for cleaning the fingers as its constant use will lead to hardening of the skin of the fingertips. We suggest that you wash your hands with soap and warm water and thoroughly dry them before pricking your finger.

23 *Will constant finger pricking make my fingers sore?*

You may find that your fingers feel sore for the first week or two after starting blood sugar monitoring but this soon disappears. We have seen many diabetics who have been measuring their blood glucose levels regularly three or four times a day for the past 5 years and who have no problems with sore fingers. Always try to rotate to different fingers.

24 *As I am a diabetic will my fingers take a long time to heal after finger pricking and am I more likely to pick up an infection of the finger?*

Your fingertips should heal as quickly as a non-diabetic but make sure you are using suitable lancets or needles (p.116). We have seen only one infected finger among many thousands of finger pricks. We suggest that you keep your hands 'socially' clean and wash them before collecting your blood sample.

25 *There are a bewildering number of blood glucose sticks and meters on the market. Which are the best to use?*

This is purely a matter of preference and may depend on the type of sticks that are most readily obtainable in your area. The sticks can be divided into two categories; those that can be read against a colour chart on the side of the bottle, and those that are best used with a meter. If you choose to use blood-testing sticks without a meter it is sensible to have someone else check how well you can read the colours as some people find this more difficult than others. A complete list of sticks and meters available in this country at time of publication is printed at the end of this section.

26 *I have recently started using BM 20-800 R test sticks but have been told that my results do not compare well with the hospital results. What is the reason for this?*

The first thing is to make sure that your technique is absolutely correct. Inaccurate results will be obtained if the correct procedures are not followed *completely* (*see* Figures 3, 4 and 5). If your technique is not at fault it could be that you are not able to interpret the colour chart correctly which can often happen. If this is so you would be advised to use a meter which reads the colour for you.

27 *My blood glucose meter appears to give slightly different results compared with the hospital laboratory. Are the meters accurate enough for daily use?*

Most results obtained when using a meter will be slightly different from the hospital laboratory results because different chemical methods are used. These slight differences do not matter and the meters are quite accurate enough for a diabetic's home use. If your results are very different from the laboratory it could be for several reasons. Firstly, is your technique correct? The most common fault is not applying a large enough drop of blood to the stick. The drop of blood must hang from the finger and look as though it is about to drop off the finger. The other fault is not applying the blood correctly on to the stick or taking too long to apply the blood to the stick. The reaction must also be timed correctly and the blood removed sufficiently, either being washed off or wiped off with cotton wool, depending on the type of stick you are using. Secondly, is your meter's stick carrier or insert kept clean? Another problem is that your sticks may be out of date. This can occur with all testing strips which if kept in a warm humid room can become inaccurate 1 month after first opening the bottle. Finally, have you read completely the instructions for using the meter and the reagent sticks? The meters and the sticks are only as accurate as the person using them.

28 *How can I tell if my meter is giving accurate answers?*

If you have any doubt about the accuracy of your meter you will be able to have some idea if you check the blood sugar level of a non-diabetic person. This should be taken before the person eats a meal and should be about 4.5 and within the range of 2.5–6.0 mmol/l. There are ways in which the accuracy of your blood tests at home can be compared with the laboratory by taking an extra drop of blood into a special tube or on to some blotting paper — this is known as Quality Control. When using Dextrostix you can also use the Ames Dextro-Chek Controls to check your performance. These are plastic vials of solutions which can be used in place of blood to perform a test. The results you obtain should fall within the values which accompany the Dextro-Chek.

*29 I have recently heard that I can cut my BM 20-800 R
sticks in half and use them like a full-width strip. What
do you advise?*

The great advantage of using BM 20-800 R strips is that they
can be cut in half longitudinally. This means that you need
less blood to apply on the pad and as these strips are
expensive it saves money. When cutting them in half it is
easier to start at the reagent-pad end and always use a sharp
pair of scissors. Medistron have recently introduced a strip
splitter which cuts the stick accurately in half and this comes
with a half-width carrier for use in the Glucocheck II meters
that use either BM 20-800 R strips or BM test BG strips (*see*
Plate 10).

Blood Testing Strips

Dextrostix by Ames. For use in a blood glucose meter.
Reads from 0–22 mmol/l. One minute test. Stick requires
washing at 60 seconds. May be used with Diagem, Gem
(Series II — Model A), Glucocheck II (Model A), Glucometer
and Hypocount A Meters. Range of readings can be
extended to 44 mmol/l by incubating with blood for only 30
seconds and multiplying the result by 2. Available in bottles
of 50 and 25, or packets of 50 and 10 foil wrapped sticks. May
be obtained from Ames, Clinitron, Hypoguard, Medistron
and Own Mumford Medical Shop. (See Figure 4).

Visidex II by Ames. For visual reading against colour
chart on the side of the bottle. Reads from 1–44 mmol/l. Two
minute test. Stick requires blotting at 30 seconds. Available
in bottles of 50 strips or packets of 20, foil wrapped strips.
Obtainable from Ames, Hypoguard or Owen Mumford
Medical Shop. (See Figure 5).

BM Test Glycemie 20-800 R by Boehringer. For visual
reading or may be used in a meter. Reads from 1–44 mmol/l
when read visually and from 2–22 mmol/l when used with a
meter. Two to three minute test. Stick requires wiping at 60
seconds. May be used with Reflolux, Glucocheck II. Range
cannot be extended by shorter incubation. Available in
bottles of 50 strips. Obtainable from Boehringer, Hypoguard,
Medistron and Owen Mumford Medical Shop. (See Figure 3).

BM Test BG Strips by Boehringer. For use in a blood glucose meter. Reads from 2–22 mmol/l. Two minute test. Stick requires wiping at 60 seconds. Range *cannot* be extended by shorter incubation. May be used with Diagem (Model B), Gem (Series II Model B), Glucocheck II (Model B) and Hypocount B meters. Available in bottles of 25 strips from Boehringer, Clinitron, Hypoguard, Medistron and Owen Mumford Medical Shop. (See Figure 3).

Blood Glucose Meters (*see* Plate 10)

Diagem Meter by Clinitron. Model A for use with Ames' Dextrostix, Model B for use with BM Test BG Strips. Operates on either mains power or rechargeable batteries. Obtainable from Clinitron or Owen Mumford Medical Shop.

Diatron Easy Test by Diatron Biomedical Instruments. Uses Diatron Easy Test reagent strips but monitor can be modified by distributor to read different strips. Has built-in memory. Operates on either mains power or disposable batteries or car lighter socket. Obtainable from Parisian Medical and Scientific.

Glucocheck II by Medistron Ltd. Three pocket size models. Model A for use with Ames' Dextrostix, Model B for use with BM Test BG Strips and Model D for use with BM Test Glycemie 20-800 R Strips. Comes complete with personal wallet, log book, pencil and instructions. Operates on disposable batteries. A strip splitter is now obtainable from Medistron Ltd, for cutting BM Test BG Strips and BM Test Glycemie 20-800 R Strips in half. This strip splitter comes complete with half-width carrier for use in the Glucocheck II. Obtainable from Medistron Ltd or Owen Mumford Medical Shop.

Glucometer by Ames. For use with Ames' Dextrostix. Comes complete with an Autolet, instruction cassette, record diary, glucose check solution and a bottle of 25 Dextrostix (the accessory pack normally costs extra except that BDA members obtain it as a special concession for the basic glucometer price). Operates on disposable batteries. Obtainable from Owen Mumford Medical Shop and Ames (large orders).

Hypo-count II by Hypoguard Ltd. Model A for use with Ames' Dextrostix and Model B for use with BM Test BG Strips. Comes complete with charger and instructions. Operates on rechargeable batteries. Obtainable from Hypoguard Ltd.

Audio Hypo-count B for Blind Diabetics by Hypoguard Ltd. Audio meter for use with BM Test BG Strips which buzzes in six different reporting blocks. Obtainable from Hypoguard Ltd.

Talking Hypo-count B for Blind Diabetics by Hypoguard Ltd. Talking meter for use with BM Test BG Strips. Uses a voice synthesizer. Obtainable from Hypoguard Ltd.

Hypo-count MX by Hypoguard Ltd. Different models for use with Ames Dextrostix or Boehringer BM strips. Has a built-in memory. Operates on a disposable battery. Obtainable from Hypoguard Ltd.

Reflocheck by Boehringer. For use with Reflocheck glucose strips and designed primarily for hospital use. Mains operated. Obtainable from Boehringer Corporation.

Reflolux by Boehringer. For use with BM Test Glycemie 20-800 R Strips. Operates on disposable batteries. Obtainable from Boehringer Corporation and Owen Mumford Medical Shop.

Finger Pricking Devices (see Plate 8)

Autolet from Owen Mumford Medical Shop. Uses either Monolet or Unilet blood lancets. Very simple operation. Obtainable from Owen Mumford Medical Shop and Medistron.

Autolet DTV From Owen Mumford Medical Shop. Uses either Monolet or Autolet blood lancets. Very simple operation. Incorporates a clock which shows the time in hours, minutes and seconds or month, date and year. This eliminates the need for a separate watch when timing reagent strips. Obtainable from Owen Mumford Medical Shop and Medistron.

Autoclix from Boehringer. For use with Monolet and Autoclix lancets. Spring-loaded lancet hidden from view during operation. Obtainable from Boehringer (large orders only) and Hypoguard.

Hemalet from Hypoguard. A slim pencil-type injector. For use with Monolet blood lancet. Obtainable from Hypoguard.

Hypoguard Finger Pricker from Hypoguard. Can be used with any disposable $\frac{1}{2}''$ or $\frac{5}{8}''$ needle. Needle hidden from view during operation. Obtainable from Hypoguard.

Mini-Lancet Small complete automatic blood lancet. Obtainable from Hypoguard.

Monojector by Monoject. For use with Monoject blood lancets. Spring-loaded lancet hidden from view during operation. Obtainable from Mariner Medical Ltd.

Auto Lancet by Genetics International. For use with Monolet blood lancets. Spring-loaded lancet hidden from view during operation. Obtainable from Genetics International.

Urine

30 I have great difficulty in becoming stabilized. I have been told to ignore my urine tests because I have a low renal threshold. Can you tell me exactly what this means?

A low renal threshold means that glucose escapes into the urine at unusually low blood glucose levels. This is particularly common during pregnancy and it occurs less frequently in other diabetics. The presence of a low renal threshold can only be established by careful comparison of simultaneous blood and urine glucose tests. If your renal threshold is low (or indeed high), then urine tests can often be misleading. There is no real way around this problem so it is clearly important that you should establish where your own renal threshold lies if you are going to rely on urine tests only as an indication of diabetic stability and control. It is because of this uncertainty in interpretation of urine tests that more and more people are finding blood glucose measurements more helpful.

31 What does it mean if I have a lot of ketones but no glucose on urine testing?

Testing for ketones in the urine can be rather confusing and unless there are special reasons for doing it, we do not normally recommend it. Some diabetics seem to develop ketones in the urine very readily, especially children, pregnant women and people who are dieting strictly to try to lose weight. Usually if glucose and ketones appear together, this indicates poor diabetic control, although as most diabetics know, this may be very transient and sugar and ketones which are present in the morning may disappear by noon. If they persist all the time then diabetic control almost certainly needs to be improved probably by increasing the insulin dose. Ketones do sometimes appear in the urine without glucose though not very frequently. It is most commonly seen in the first morning specimen and probably occurs as the insulin action from the night before is wearing off: it occurs because in some people the ketone levels increase before the glucose levels. Under these circumstances it is not serious and no particular action is needed. Occasionally, however, this may be an indication of night-time hypoglycaemia which can go undetected. If this is at all likely you should check your blood glucose at 3.00 a.m. on several occasions to see how low it goes. Lastly, ketones without glucose in the urine are very common in people who are trying to lose weight through calorie restriction. Anyone who is on a strict diet and losing weight will burn up body fat which causes ketones to appear in the urine. Provided there is not excess sugar in the urine (or the blood), these ketones do not mean that the diabetes is out of control.

32 When ketones and glucose are present in the urine at the same time, what does this indicate?

When this occurs in only one sample of urine and is gone by the next one, it indicates some slight imbalance in diabetic control. If on the other hand the ketones and glucose are present in a series of urine samples passed one after the other and accompanied by increasing thirst and tendency to make urine, then they are an indication that the diabetic control is severely out of balance and may be followed by diabetic ketoacidosis. In this case you should contact your doctor urgently.

33   My son tests his urine once a week. Is this enough or should he do his tests more frequently?

Only one test a week is not really anything like enough and is of little value. The number of tests to be done per day depends a lot on stability of control. When one is starting treatment for the first time or when some illness has upset diabetic control, there is no substitute for testing every sample of urine that is passed until control has been achieved. If this is not possible then check a sample of urine before each main meal and before going to bed and continue this until the balance is restored. These four times of testing are most useful because they tend to reflect the peaks and troughs of blood glucose control. When testing is carried out in a well-stabilized patient we recommend that these four time points are still used and that each patient should endeavour to complete two tests at each of those points each week. This can either be in the form of 2 days in which a full profile test is made, or the tests are done in such a way that at the end of each week there are two results available for each testing time. These records should be kept in a neat and orderly way so that they can be shown to your medical adviser and discussed in relationship to your treatment.

People are increasingly going over from urine testing to blood testing. The same guidelines are recommended with the addition that many diabetics find it very helpful to do occasional glood glucose readings at 3.00 a.m. to detect hypoglycaemia even if this means setting the alarm clock to wake them up! This does not need to be done throughout life but only at times when the balance becomes unstable.

34   I have been stabilized on a mixture of slow- and fast-acting insulins which I inject once daily before breakfast. Blood tests have shown that my glucose levels before breakfast and after lunch are good but I am concerned about the mid-morning one. The urine tests I take at mid-morning are invariably positive, showing ¾-1% (+ + to + + +) yet this after-meal peak does not occur after lunch or dinner. Does the positive result matter?

You have made an observation about diabetic control which doctors and nurses notice frequently — mid-morning blood and urine tests tend to be on the high side. It is not always easy to eliminate this but here are a few suggestions:

a   You should allow 10–15 minutes between the insulin injection and breakfast to ensure some absorption of the short-acting insulin to cover breakfast.
b   You might need more quick and less slow-acting insulin.
c   You might need to take a smaller breakfast and in compensation a larger lunch.
d   For the very best control you might find it better to be treated with two injections. This is often the ideal solution offering not only the best control but also the greatest flexibility.

Finally, if mid-morning is the only time you show sugar in the urine, this may indicate that your control is usually rather good but you should be guided by the more accurate haemoglobin A_1 measurement (p.129) which your General Practitioner or Diabetic Clinic may be able to measure.

35   *Why do we not always get a true blood sugar through a urine test (as in my case)?*

In most people urine only contains glucose when the glucose concentration in the blood is higher than a certain figure (usually 10 mmol/l). So below this level urine tests give no indication at all to the concentration of glucose in the blood. The level at which glucose spills into the urine (renal threshold) (p.126) varies from one diabetic to another and you can only assess it in yourself by making many simultaneous blood and urine glucose measurements. If you undertake this exercise you will undoubtedly find like most other people that the relationship between the blood and urine glucose concentrations is not very precise; for this reason most diabetics nowadays prefer to do blood tests rather than urine tests since they find that the increased precision of blood tests outweighs any disadvantage that may stem from having to prick your finger to get a drop of blood.

36 My urine tests nearly always show orange (+ + + +, greater than 2%) but my clinic tells me that my blood glucose is low. How can I learn about what state my glucose is in?

It sounds as if your renal threshold (p.129) is low. You will probably find that blood glucose monitoring is more satisfactory to help you maintain your balance. It would certainly be worth your while to undertake a number of simultaneous blood and urine tests so that you can see for yourself how well (or how badly) they relate to each other If you do have a low renal threshold and have 2% in the urine when the blood glucose is less than 5 or 6 mmol/l, then urine tests do not tell you anything useful and you should stop doing them. Blood tests are absolutely necessary for people with a low renal threshold who wish to control their diabetes.

37 Can you please inform me what 2% (+ + + +) glucose in the urine means in the form of carbohydrates and what amount of insulin is required to be injected to cancel out 2% glucose in the urine?

This is a common question and the first thing to be said is that there is no direct answer. It is a mistake to think that once you have found a high test you can treat that test by giving yourself a dose of insulin which is related to the value of the test. You are asked to do tests on a regular basis so that you and your medical advisers can help to identify a pattern in the urine tests (or blood tests) that over a period of time (usually a week or so) indicate the balance of your control. If there is a regular pattern such as continued 2% sugar before lunch and reasonable tests at other times of the day, then this would indicate the need for either more insulin in the morning to cover breakfast or a smaller breakfast. The actual amount by which you increase your morning injection or decrease the amount of carbohydrate you have at breakfast is to a certain extent a matter of trial and error. In the first instance we would suggest increasing your insulin dose by 4 units (2 units if dose less than 12 units) or by reducing the carbohydrate content of the meal by 10 grams. If these measures are insufficient it is easy to make a further adjustment. It is better to err on the side of a small adjustment rather than to be too dramatic and expose yourself to the risk of hypoglycaemia.

38 How do you know if you have ketones in your urine? What are they and are they dangerous?

You test urine for ketones with either Ketostix, Ketodiastix or Acetest tablets. Ketones are breakdown products of fat stores of the body which are present in small amounts even in non-diabetic persons particularly when they are dieting or fasting and therefore relying on their body fat stores for energy fuel. In diabetics small amounts of ketones in the urine are commonly found. They become dangerous only when they are present in large amounts. This is usually associated with a severe disturbance in diabetic control, usually accompanied by thirst, passing large amounts of urine, and nausea. If the ketones are in the urine together with continuous 2% (+ + + +) glucose then they are dangerous since this is the condition which precedes the development of diabetic ketoacidosis and under these circumstances you should seek urgent medical advice.

39 If you are testing urine four times a day, is it necessary to empty the bladder each time before the test? In my experience this is easier said than done

The 'double voiding' technique that you describe is not essential for every test and we agree with your comments. It is only necessary if many hours have elapsed since the previous bladder emptying which in practice means the first morning specimen only, otherwise it is only required if one is attempting to compare blood glucose tests with urine tests.

40   At what time of day should I test my urine? I am on diet only

If your first test in the morning before breakfast is continually negative as it should be if you are on diet only, you can test your urine occasionally before lunch, before your evening meal or at bedtime, and you should find it negative at these times. If these are all negative you should try checking it 2–3 hours after breakfast which is the most likely time when you will find glucose in the urine. If this is negative too then there is nothing further that you can do to monitor your control more accurately by urine tests. You should check that your fasting blood glucose values are 6 mmol/l or less and that your routine haemoglobin A_1 measurement is less than 8.5%. If you can achieve these goals then by all criteria your diabetes is exceptionally well controlled and you are to be congratulated.

41   For some time now I have suffered from diabetes. I am always curious to know what type of tests are made with my urine specimen when they are taken off into the laboratory

Urine specimens are tested for three things, glucose, ketones and albumin (protein). These tests serve only as a spot check and are meant to complement your own tests performed at home. Clinics like to know the percentage of sugar taken at different times of day as giving some measure of control at home. The detection of ketones is of rather limited value since some patients make ketones very easily and others almost not at all. The presence of protein in the urine can indicate either infection in the urine or the presence of some kidney disease and in diabetics this is likely to be diabetic nephropathy, one of the long-standing diabetic complications (p.245).

42   I have a strong family history of diabetes. My daughter recently tested her urine and found 2% glucose. However, her blood glucose was only 8 mmol/l. She underwent a glucose tolerance test and this was normal.

Could she have diabetes or could there be another reason why she is passing glucose in her water?

It is very unlikely that she has diabetes if a glucose tolerance test was normal. If she had glucose in the urine during the glucose tolerance test at which time all the blood glucose readings were strictly normal, then this would indicate that she has a low renal threshold for glucose (p.117). If this is the correct diagnosis then it is important to find out whether she passes glucose in her urine first thing in the morning while fasting or only after she has eaten. In people who pass glucose in the urine during the fasting state, there is not known to be any increased incidence of development of diabetes and the condition (renal glycosuria) is strongly inherited. If on the other hand she only passes glucose in the urine after meals containing starch and sugar, this condition sometimes progresses to diabetes.

43 What is the difference between a urine test using two drops of urine instead of five drops of urine?

When the blood glucose is very high, glucose can pass into the urine in large amounts such that the concentration can under some circumstances become as high as 20g/100ml (20%). When this urine is tested with either Clinitest or Diastix it will just record a value which is greater than 2% (+ + + + +). The range of the Clinitest tablets can be extended from 2% to 10% when only two drops of urine are taken rather than five drops of urine, an orange test with two drops of urine indicating 10% or more glucose in the urine. In fact if you take only one drop of urine instead of five drops of urine you can extend the range even further. Under these circumstances an orange test will only be seen when the urine contains 20 g glucose/100 ml. This method of urine testing certainly increases the range of measurement but does not improve the accuracy of the relationship between the blood and urine tests. The only way of getting a more accurate estimation of blood glucose is to measure it directly.

44 When are the best times to do a urine test?

This depends largely on the reason for wanting to do the test. Firstly if you have lost control of your diabetes and are trying to re-establish it you should test every urine sample that you pass until things are back to normal. If your diabetes is just mildly out of control and you think there is room for improvement then the best times for test are immediately before the morning injection (this should be a 'double voided' specimen), secondly immediately before lunch, thirdly immediately before supper and fourthly before retiring to bed (also a double-voided specimen). You should make these regular measurements for 4 days and look for a pattern in the results (e.g. consistently between $\frac{1}{2}$ and 2% before the evening meal). Only when you establish a pattern should you take steps to try to improve control. Once you are well balanced and just want to check that things are on an even keel, you should use the same times (i.e. before main meals and before bed) to try to do two tests at each of these points every week — though not necessarily on the same days. These routine 'tests' show when balance is slipping in time to make adjustments before things get badly out of control.

45 Many doctors seem to prefer negative urine tests. I encourage my son to ensure that there is a low glucose level in his urine. What is the ideal test?

Doctors prefer to see negative urine tests because it is only under these circumstances that they can be sure that blood glucose is close to normal which is everyone's goal in therapy. You undoubtedly encourage your son to show the presence of some glucose in his urine to reduce the risk of hypoglycaemic attacks. Unfortunately this attitude is potentially dangerous in the long term because although you may avoid the short-term problems with hypoglycaemia you expose your son to the longer term risks of diabetic complications (retinopathy, neuropathy, nephropathy) which develop gradually over many years as a result of persistently high blood glucose levels. In answer to the last part of your question, the ideal test is to measure blood glucose and not to rely on urine tests. Unfortunately, blood cannot be obtained without pricking a finger.

46 *I always show ketones, often quite heavily, in my morning urine test although the glucose is negative. I never show ketones at any other time. Why is this?*

The presence of ketones in the early morning urine test reflects the fact that your body has been relying on its stored fat to provide a large proportion of the energy required in the night and this is perfectly normal. One often finds ketones when doing urine tests in the morning even in non-diabetic persons, particularly children. There is no need at all to worry about this.

47 *I am a diabetic controlled by tablets and the urine checks I make invariably turn out to be negative. However, the blood glucose tests taken in the clinic turn out to be surprisingly high, even as high as 16, at the same time as my negative urine tests. Why is this?*

You are describing quite clearly what is known as a high renal threshold. This means that in your case glucose tests in the urine are of little value. It does not indicate that you have abnormal kidneys but it does suggest that you would be better off learning how to do blood glucose tests. It is the high blood glucose which over the years may cause complications, and the negative urine tests in the presence of a high blood glucose may be very misleading.

48 *If my urine tests are regularly blue (negative) can my blood sugar levels be high?*

Yes, they can. It all depends on where your renal threshold lies, i.e. at what blood glucose level you begin to pass glucose in the urine. The best way of checking on this is to do a series of simultaneous blood and urine samples over a period of several weeks and find out for yourself what level of glucose in the blood you begin to find glucose in the urine. Having once discovered this 'renal threshold' it tends to stay constant for many years. Having once done the comparison between blood and urine tests you will know approximately your blood glucose values from the urine test result. You may find like many patients that having done these simultaneous blood and urine tests you would rather continue in the future with the blood test.

49 *A colleague has asked me whether all diabetics should be tested for colour blindness in case this might impair their ability to test urine*

You draw attention to a real and not uncommon problem. Twenty per cent (one in five) of males are affected by some form of red/green colour blindness and it has been shown that this impairs their ability to read the results of urine tests, and probably the same problem applies also to reading sticks used for blood testing. There is another form of colour blindness that affects both males and females who have diabetic retinopathy and it has also been shown that this form of colour blindness also impairs the ability to read colours on the urine sticks and probably the blood sticks. We do not recommend the routine testing of all diabetics for colour blindness but when they are being taught either blood or urine monitoring their ability to read the colours accurately should be checked by the person (doctor or nurse) who is instructing them.

50 *I have recently started showing 2% sugar in my urine tests. My doctor tells me that as I am feeling well I should stop doing the urine tests as they are invalid. Is there any reason why I should test my urine?*

You should undoubtedly continue to test the urine and the advice you have had seems rather suspect unless your doctor knows more than you convey in your question (perhaps you have a very low renal threshold for glucose). It is quite possible for urine tests to be constantly 2% without there being obvious symptoms but with a very high blood glucose level. This means that you are unnecessarily exposing yourself to risks of developing long-term diabetic complications. Even though you are feeling well it is imperative at all times to maintain the best control that is possible. If your doctor is correct in saying that your own particular urine tests are invalid, then this is an indication for doing blood testing rather than no testing at all.

51 *My son tested his urine with my Clinitest and found the result positive. However, his GP told him that alcohol affects tests and he should take no notice of them as he had drunk four pints of beer before testing. Is this true?*

No. Alcohol does not affect the urine test itself, neither does it make the blood sugar unduly high in a non-diabetic person. It sounds as if your son should be further investigated with blood sugars and possibly a glucose tolerance test to find out whether he has or has not got diabetes.

52 *My husband is an insulin-requiring diabetic and is fanatical about keeping his urine test blue. As a result he has some severe hypos. How serious would it be if his tests were occasionally green and would this reduce the risk of hypos?*

Your husband is aiming to achieve and maintain very good diabetic control, and it is right that he should do so. However, it is obviously tiresome if as a result he suffers a lot of hypos. This situation could be dealt with in two ways. If the hypos always occur at the same time each day he could increase his carbohydrate portions at the preceding meal or snack. If, on the other hand, the hypos occur randomly at any time of the day or night then he needs to reduce his insulin dose a little. If as a result some of his tests become slightly positive for glucose this would be preferable to having frequent severe hypos. An alternative strategy that your husband needs to consider is to see if he can improve his balance by using blood tests rather than urine tests.

*53 I do not understand why it is that glucose from the
    blood only spills into the urine above a certain level; I
    gather this level is known as the 'renal threshold' —
    could you explain it for me in a little more detail?*

Urine is formed by filtration of blood in the kidneys. When
the glucose concentration in the blood is below about 10
mmol/l, any glucose filtered into the urine is subsequently re-
absorbed into the body. When the level of glucose exceeds
approximately 10 mmol/l ('the renal threshold') more glucose
is filtered than the body can re-absorb and the result is that
it is passed in the urine. Once the level has exceeded 10
mmol/l, the amount of glucose in the urine will be
proportional to the level of glucose in the blood. Below 10
mmol/l, however, there will be no glucose in the urine and
since in non-diabetics blood glucose level never exceeds 10
mmol/l, a non-diabetic has no glucose in his urine.

Haemoglobin A_1

*54 What is haemoglobin A_1 and what are the normal
    values?*

Haemoglobin A_1 (HbA_1) is a component of the red pigment
(haemoglobin A; HbA) present in the blood to carry oxygen
from the lungs to the various organs in the body. Using a
variety of laboratory methods the HbA_1 can be measured as
a percentage of all the haemoglobin present. HbA_1 consists
of HbA combined with glucose by a chemical link. The
amount of HbA_1 present is directly proportional to the
average blood glucose during the 120-day life span of the
HbA-containing red blood corpuscles in the circulating blood.
    It is a relatively new test only now becoming widely
available which is the most successful of all the tests so far
developed to give an index of goodness (or badness) of
diabetic control. Blood glucose tests which we have used for
many years fluctuate too erratically with injections, meals
and other events for an isolated sample taken at the clinic
visit to give much information about the degree of diabetic
control since the last clinic visit. HbA_1 averages out all the

peaks and troughs of the blood glucose over the previous 2–3 months before the test is done. This is of great advantage to yourself and to your doctor because if the value is normal, you know that you are doing well and need not struggle to do better. On the other hand, if the value is high it indicates that overall control is poor and that new avenues of treatment need to be explored.

The normal values vary a little from laboratory to laboratory but in a non-diabetic person HbA$_1$ values usually run between 6 and 8.5%. In a poorly controlled diabetic, or one who has only recently been diagnosed the values can go as high as 20 or 25% which reflects a consistently high average blood glucose over the preceding 2–3 months. On the other hand, in somebody who has perfect control, blood sugars averaging in the normal range, the HbA$_1$ will be in the range of 6–8.5% and in the occasional patient who runs their blood sugars too low due to taking too much insulin, then the values will actually be sub-normal, below 6%.

55   How often need it be done?

Because it averages the blood glucose levels over a 2–3 month interval there is no point in doing this test often (say every 3 months) unless the values are very high and one is trying to improve control. If the values are normal and control is satisfactory 2–4 measurements per year should be sufficient.

56   My blood tests that I do at home with my BM20-800 R strips are all normal (less than 10 mmol/l). When I went to the diabetic clinic they told me that my HbA$_1$ was very high (15%) and that this was not consistent with the blood sugar reading I had made at home — why is this?

It sounds as if there is an error in your reading of the BM sticks and that your true blood sugar readings are higher than you think they are. An HbA$_1$ of 15% suggests that your blood sugar averages more than 10 mmol/l. You need to check the accuracy of your blood sugar monitoring.

57 *I am 25 years old and have had diabetes since I was 15. I
have been attending the clinic regularly every 3 months
and do regular blood sugar tests at home with my own
meter. At my last clinic visit the doctor I saw said he
did not need to see me again for a whole year because
my HbA_1 was consistently normal — why did he do
this?*

It sounds as though your specialist has tremendous
confidence in you and your ability to control your diabetes.
As long as you can keep it this way he clearly feels that
seeing you once a year is sufficient. He can then spend more
time with those other patients who are not as successful as
yourself. You should feel very proud of this.

58 *I am a mild diabetic treated only by diet. I find it very
difficult to stick to my diet or do the tests between my
clinic visits but I am always very strict for the few days
before I am seen at the clinic and my blood glucose test
is usually normal. At my last clinic visit my blood
glucose was 5 mmol/l but the doctor said he was very
unhappy about my diabetic control because the HbA_1
was too high at 12% — what did he mean?*

Your experience shows very nicely the usefulness of HbA_1
testing, because quite clearly you have been misleading
yourself as well as your medical advisers about your ability
to cope with your diabetes. The HbA_1 test has brought this
to the surface for the first time. Because the HbA_1 reflects
what your blood glucose has been doing for as long as 2
months before your clinic visit, your last-minute attempts to
get your diabetes under control before you went to the clinic
were enough to bring the blood glucose down but the HbA_1
still remained high.

59 *I have had diabetes treated with insulin for more than
20 years now and have always troubled to keep myself
as well controlled as possible, initially using urine tests
to balance myself, more recently with blood tests. I am
never satisfied that I have things under control since
my blood sugar is always swinging up and down and*

*never stays steady like my husband's when I do his (he
is not diabetic). At the last clinic visit a specialist said
that my HbA$_1$ was normal at 7% and he was completely
happy with the way I am looking after myself — how
can this be true?*

Although your blood sugar is swinging up and down more
than your husband's, the fact that your HbA$_1$ is 7% means
that your blood sugar on average is normal. If you are not
having troublesome hypos (I presume from your question
you are not) then it sounds as if you have achieved as good
control as is possible and deserve to be congratulated.

60 *My recent HbA$_1$ was said to be low at 6%. Blood sugar
    readings look all right, on average about 5 mmol/l. The
    specialist asked me to set the alarm clock and check
    some at 3 o'clock in the morning — why is this?*

A low HbA$_1$ suggests that at some stage your blood sugars
are running unduly low. If you are not having hypoglycaemic
attacks during the day then it is possible they are occurring
at night and you are sleeping through them. By doing 3.00
a.m. blood glucose tests you should be able to determine
whether this is so.

61 *My diabetes is treated with diet and glibenclamide
    tablets. By strict dieting I have lost weight down to
    slightly below my target figure and all my urine tests
    are negative. My HbA$_1$ test I am told is still too high at
    11% and does not seem to be falling despite the fact
    that I am still losing weight. I cannot be any stricter
    with what I eat. At the last clinic visit the doctor said
    that I am going to have to go on to insulin injections. I
    have been dreading these all my life — is he right?*

It sounds very much as if you have reached the stage where
diet and tablets aren't strong enough to keep your diabetes
properly under control and even in the absence of any sugar
in your urine a consistently high HbA$_1$ indicates that your
blood sugar is running too high and that you need to move on
to the next stronger form of treatment which is insulin

injection. You have been given sound advice and I am sure it will not turn out to be as bad as you imagine and you will feel a great deal better which will make it all worth while.

62 *At my last visit to the hospital diabetic clinic they told me that I had an abnormal haemoglobin but that it was nothing to worry about and then went on to ask me if my ancestors came from near the Mediterranean, which is true — how did they know that and what does it all mean?*

At the time that you had your HbA$_1$ measured they were probably able to detect the presence of another component in your blood which is common in some countries, particularly those around the Mediterranean. This is usually present in such small amounts that it does not do any harm and it sounds as if this is what is happening in your case.

Diabetic Clinic

63 *They have just appointed a new young consultant at my hospital and I am told that they are going to start a special diabetic clinic — will this offer any advantage to me?*

Most hospitals these days have at least one of the senior doctors who specializes in diabetes and by running a special diabetic clinic can bring together all the specially trained doctors, nurses, dietitians and chiropodists and this should mean a better service for you and other diabetics attending the clinic. You will have the benefit of seeing people who have special training in diabetes, and most patients find this a big advantage.

64 *My GP is starting a diabetic clinic in the local group practice and tells me that I no longer need to attend the hospital clinic. It's much more convenient for me to go to see my GP but will this be all right?*

You are very fortunate that your general practitioner clearly has a special interest in diabetes and has gone to the trouble of setting up a special clinic in the practice for this. Quite a lot of GPs have had special training in diabetes and it is becoming quite fashionable to set up these general-practice-based 'mini-diabetic clinics'. I am sure your hospital specialist will know about this. If you have any anxieties why not discuss it with him, he may even attend the mini-clinic from time to time.

65   *Although they do a blood test every time I go to our local diabetic clinic they now only test the urine once a year when they look at my eyes and check my blood pressure — why is this?*

With the introduction of HbA_1 measurement and blood glucose monitoring the value of urine testing is really for the detection of proteinuria (albumin) as an indicator of possible kidney damage. This doesn't need to be done more often than once a year in people who are quite well and free from albumin in their urine. As a general rule all diabetics should have their urine, eyes and blood pressure checked annually.

66   *Why do I have to wait such a long time every time I go to the diabetic clinic?*

If you think about it, you probably have quite a lot of tests done and it takes time to get the answers back and the results all together before you see the doctor. This is particularly likely to be so if you have a blood glucose and the HbA_1 levels measured in the clinic which take time to process. Although it may be irritating to have to wait for these results, they are very important as they can be used in a two-way discussion between you and the doctor to review your control and progress with diabetes. Many clinics use this waiting time for showing educational films or videos about diabetes and for meeting the dietitian and/or the chiropodist.

67   *What determines whether my next appointment is in 1 month or 6 months?*

Generally speaking, if your control is consistently good you will not need to be seen very often; on the other hand, if your control if poor it is likely that you will be seen more often. This is not, as you might perhaps think, a subtle form of punishment but it will give both of you more opportunity to sort out what is going wrong.

68 *At my clinic we have a mixture of patients from young children to very old pensioners — why do they not have special clinics for young people?*

Although it may be desirable to have a special clinic for younger patients it may not always be possible with the limited resources of the Health Service or a given hospital. Some people would feel that it may not even be desirable and that all patients in the clinic are united by the fact that they have diabetes. Certainly from the point of view of clinic organization there is no difference between the young children and the pensioners. The principles of diabetes care are common throughout all ages.

69 *We have a specialist nurse in diabetes working in the diabetic clinic that I attend. What does she do?*

Many clinics in this country now employ specialist nurses who spend their whole time working with diabetic patients. They may work in the community and/or the hospital and have a variety of titles — Diabetic Health Visitor, Diabetic Community Nurse, Diabetic or Diabetes Liaison Nurse, Diabetes Nurse Specialist, Diabetic Sister, Diabetes or Diabetic Care Sister, etc. These senior nurses spend most of their time educating patients, giving advice (much of it on the telephone), making decisions about patient management and teaching other members of the medical and nursing staff about diabetes. They are experts in their field and are very valuable members of the diabetic team.

Eyes — see also p.236

70 I have just been discovered to have diabetes and the glasses that I have had for years seem no longer suitable but my doctor tells me not to get them changed until my diabetes has been brought under control — is this right?

Yes. When the sugar concentration in the body rises this affects the focusing ability of the eyes but it is only a temporary effect and things go back to normal once the sugar has been brought under control. If you change your glasses now you will be able to see better but as soon as your diabetes is brought under control you will need to change them yet again so it is best to delay making a decision, as to whether you need a new pair of glasses, until your diabetes has been controlled for at least a month.

71 Why do I have to have my eyes checked regularly every year as a diabetic?

As you have undoubtedly heard, after many years diabetes can affect the retina (back of the eye) and the routine eye checks are aimed at picking this up at the early stage before it seriously affects your vision and at a stage where it can be effectively treated.

72 As a diabetic how often should I have my eyes tested? I do not need glasses; my vision, as far as I can see, is completely normal

Check this with your specialist but if your diabetes is well controlled and your vision is normal and you have no diabetic changes, then once a year is generally sufficient.

73 When I was at the diabetic clinic last time the specialist there said to me that it was my responsibility to make sure that my eyes were checked every year — who shall I get to do this?

I am sure your specialist was just reminding you that it is desirable for all patients to have their eyes checked annually. This can be done by either the specialist in the diabetic clinic, the specialist in the eye clinic, the local general practitioner if he feels that he is sufficiently well trained to do this, or your local ophthalmic optician if he feels able to do it. You need to undergo two examinations. One is to test your 'visual acuity' — which is basically the ability to read those letters on the chart down to the right line — and the second is to have the back of your eyes looked at with an ophthalmoscope; this is the more difficult of the two examinations and can only be done by somebody with special training. If you have any doubts as to whom should check your eyes discuss it with your specialist.

74 *Last time I was up at the clinic when they were checking my eyes on the chart with the letters on, they made me look through a small pin-hole and to my surprise, I could see much better and read letters on the line two down from the one that I could see without the pin-hole — why was this?*

This indicates that you need spectacles for distant vision. For example, you are probably having trouble reading the numbers on the buses and this will be improved with a pair of distance glasses. The pin-hole acts as a universal correcting lens.

75 *Why do they put drops in your eyes at the clinic that sting, enlarge the pupil and blur the vision?*

These make it much easier for the doctor examining the back of your eye with an ophthalmoscope. It is sometimes not possible to examine the eye properly without dilating the pupil to get a clearer view.

76 *At my last clinic visit they warned me that at the next visit they were going to put drops in my eyes to dilate the pupil and that I should plan not to drive for 24 hours after the clinic visit — why is this?*

The drops that are used to dilate the pupil so that the doctor can get a good look at the back of your eye also paralyse the lens that allows your sight to focus properly. The effects of the drops may last as long as 24 hours and this may impair your vision sufficiently to make you unsafe at the wheel — better not to take any risks.

77 *I have had diabetes for 20 years and seem to be quite well. When the doctor looked in my eyes last time I saw him, he said he could see some mild diabetic changes and referred me to a special clinic called Retinopathy Clinic — what does this mean; am I about to go blind?*

There is no need for alarm. It would be surprising if after 20 years of diabetes it was not possible for him to find some changes in the eye. He probably considers it appropriate that you should be seen by an eye specialist and maybe have some special photographs taken of the eyes in order to examine them in more detail and to be of use for future reference.

78 *What is retinopathy?*

Retinopathy is a condition affecting the back of the eye (the retina) which may occur in long-standing diabetics, particularly those in whom control has not been very good. There is a gradual development of abnormalities of the blood flow to the back of the eye which can lead to deterioration of vision as a result of either disturbance of the function of the eye itself, or as a result of bleeding into the eye from the abnormal blood vessels. Retinopathy is usually easily diagnosed by examination of the eye by an expert with an ophthalmoscope, and it can usually be picked up a long time before it leads to any disturbance in vision. Treatment at this stage with laser usually arrests the process and slows or stops further deterioration. Annual eye checks are carried out in order to pick up retinopathy at a stage before it causes significant upset in vision and ensures that treatment is carried out as soon as it is appropriate.

79 *What are cataracts?*

Cataracts are the changes that occur in the lens of the eye leading to gradual loss of transparency and eventually interfering with vision, by interfering with the transmission of light into the eye. Cataracts occur in non-diabetics as well as diabetics and are generally considered to be a normal effect of ageing. There is some evidence to suggest that they may occur at a slightly earlier age in diabetics than non-diabetics. They are often present for many years before they lead to any significant interference with vision, and when vision does become reduced, as a result of cataracts, it can usually be dramatically improved by removal of the cataracts and the fitting of a suitable lens. There is also a very rare form of cataract (snowstorm cataract) which occurs in young children who have particularly bad control over the first few years of their diabetes.

80 What is laser treatment?

Laser treatment is a form of treatment with a pencil of light used to cause very small burns on the back of the eye (retina). It is used in the treatment of many eye conditions including diabetic retinopathy. The laser burns are created in the bits of the retina not used for detailed vision, sparing the important areas required for reading, etc. This form of treatment has been shown to arrest or delay the progress of diabetic retinopathy, provided that it is given at a sufficiently early stage before useful vision is lost and in adequate amounts. It is sometimes necessary to give small doses of laser treatment intermittently over many years; occasionally it can all be dealt with over a relatively short period. The eyes need continuous assessment thereafter, since it is possible that further treatment may be needed at any stage.

Chiropody and foot care — see also p.241

81 I have just developed diabetes and have been warned that as a diabetic I am much more likely to get into trouble with my feet and need to take great care of them — what does this mean?

As long as you keep your diabetes well controlled and have no loss of sensation in your feet and good circulation to your feet then you are no more at risk than a non-diabetic. In the long term there is a suggestion that diabetics are more prone to foot trouble and it pays to get into good habits — inspecting the feet, keeping the nails properly trimmed and avoiding ill-fitting shoes right from the outset. As a diabetic you usually have access to the local chiropodist who will check your feet and advise you on any questions that you may have.

82   *I have had diabetes for 10 years and as far as I can see it is quite under control and I am told that I am free from complications, but I cannot help worrying about the possibility of developing gangrene in the feet — can you tell me what it is and what causes it?*

Gangrene is death of tissues in any part of the body. It most commonly occurs in the toes and fingers. Gangrene also occurs in non-diabetics and diabetics are prone to it only if they have serious impairment of blood supply to their feet or loss of sensation. If the major blood vessels get clogged up then this can lead to gangrene and the main cause of this is smoking; generally it occurs only in older people and is related to the progressive hardening of the arteries that is part of the ageing process. The other form of gangrene that can occur in diabetics is that due to the presence of infection which usually affects the feet in people who have lost sensation because of diabetic neuropathy. This can occur even in the presence of good blood supply. Any ulcer or infection affecting the feet must be treated promptly and seriously, and if you see anything on your feet which you are worried about you should consult your doctor without delay.

83   *As a diabetic do I have to take any special precautions when cutting my toenails?*

Only if the sensation in your feet is impaired. If this is the case you need to be very careful not to damage your toes which could act as a focus for infection.

84   *I have a thick callus on the top of one of my toes — can I use a corn plaster on this?*

If sensation and circulation in your feet are quite normal you can use a corn plaster with care but it would be safer to consult a chiropodist to have it treated.

85   *My son has picked up athletes' foot, allegedly from the swimming pool at school. He is a diabetic treated with insulin — do I have to take any special precautions about using the powder and cream given to me by my doctor?*

No. Athletes' foot is very common and is due to a fungal infection and should respond briskly to treatment with the appropriate antibiotic plus the usual precautions of keeping the feet clean and drying them carefully.

86   *Does diabetes cause bunions?*

No. Bunions are no more common in diabetics than non-diabetics.

87   *I have had diabetes for 25 years and I have been warned that the sensation in my feet is not normal. I am troubled with an ingrowing toenail on my great toe which often gets red but does not hurt — what shall I do about it?*

You should seek help and advice *urgently* because you are particularly vulnerable to the infection spreading without you being aware of the seriousness of it because it does not hurt as much as it would in someone with normal sensation.

88   *I am 67, had diabetes for 15 years and seem to be fit and well and as far as I can ascertain my feet are quite healthy. My vision is not as good as it used to be and I find it quite difficult to inspect my feet carefully — what can I do about it?*

Do you have a friend or relative who can inspect your feet regularly for you and trim the nails? If you have anxiety or if this is not possible then the sensible thing to do would be to attend a chiropodist, either locally or at your diabetic clinic for regular inspection.

89   Do I have to pay for chiropody?

Most hospital diabetic departments provide a chiropody service free of charge. Outside the hospital service, chiropody under the National Health Service is limited to pensioners, pregnant women and schoolchildren; although local rules do vary and some enterprising districts do make free chiropody available to diabetics. It is prudent, therefore, to make some local enquiries before paying any money!

90   Can you give me a simple list of rules for foot care?

If you are young with normal vision and have no loss of sensation in your feet or impairment of blood supply to your feet then you really need to take no more care of your feet than non-diabetics. It is only when there is either loss of blood supply to the feet or, more particularly, loss of sensation that you have to be particularly careful about the care to your feet. It is therefore essential that you are aware of what your doctor considers to be the current status of your feet.

The list of foot rules that follows is aimed specifically for those who have abnormalities of either blood supply or neuropathy. If you have any impairment of your vision then you should get somebody else with good eyesight to help you in your regular inspection and care of your feet.

Foot Care Rules

Do   Wash feet daily with soap and *warm* water. Do not use hot water.

Do   Dry feet well with a soft towel, especially between the toes.

Do   Change socks or stockings daily.

Do   Wear comfortable shoes — *not* too tight or too loose.

Do	Cut toenails across, following the shape of the end of the toe, *not* deep into the corners. This is easier after bathing.
Do	Check your feet daily when bathing and see your doctor about any foot problems.
Do	See a chiropodist if in any doubt about foot care, e.g. nails and corns.
Do not	Put your feet on hot water bottles or sit too close to a fire or radiator.
Do not	Use corn paints or plasters or attempt to cut your own corns with knives or razors under any circumstances.
Do not	Wear tight garters. Wear a suspender belt or tights instead.
Do not	Wear new shoes for long periods to 'break them in'.
Do not	Walk barefoot.
Do not	Let feet get dry and cracked. Use hand lotion to keep skin soft.
Do not	Cut the toenails too short.

Seek advice immediately if you notice:
  Any colour change in your leg or foot.
  Any discharge from a break or crack in the skin, or from a corn or from beneath a toenail.
  Any swelling or throbbing in any part of your foot.

First Aid Measures

Minor injuries can be treated at home provided professional help is sought if the injury does not respond quickly to first aid. Minor cuts and abrasions should be cleaned gently with cotton wool or gauze and then a modern antiseptic, such as Savlon or cetrimide cream should be applied. Clean gauze should be lightly bandaged in place. If blisters occur, do not prick them. If they burst dress them as a minor cut. Never use strong medicaments such as iodine. Never place adhesive strapping directly over a wound. Always apply gauze first.

Brittle diabetes

91 What is 'brittle diabetes' and what treatment does it require?

The term 'brittle diabetes' is applied to an insulin-treated diabetic who oscillates from one extreme to the other, i.e. from severe hyperglycaemia (blood sugar much too high) to severe hypoglycaemia with all the problems that are encountered in a 'hypo'. A diabetic with this problem is frequently admitted to hospital for 'restabilization'. The term 'brittle' is not a good one because to some extent the blood sugar of all diabetics taking insulin swings during the 24 hours from high to low and back again. The term 'brittle' is therefore restricted to those diabetics in whom the swings of blood sugar are sufficiently serious to cause inconvenience with or without admission to hospital. It is important to realize that 'brittle diabetes' is *not* a special type of diabetes and only applies when the instability is severe. This normally occurs at a time when maybe a diabetic may be emotionally unsettled. It is therefore particularly common amongst teenagers, especially girls. It is most encouraging that as emotional stability and maturity are reached so 'brittle diabetes' disappears and most of these patients will become reasonably stable and frequent admissions to hospital cease. During any particularly difficult period it is well worth remembering that it will not last for ever.

92 I am a 'brittle diabetic' and my doctor has advised me to stop working — what does this mean and am I entitled to Social Security Benefit?

The term 'brittle diabetes' is used rather too loosely. It is usually taken to mean someone whose blood sugar rises or falls very quickly and the patient may develop unexpected hypos. Many conditions may contribute to this but one of the most common factors is an excessive or inappropriate insulin dosage. Other factors which may contribute include irregular meals and life-style, poor injection techniques and general ignorance about the problems of balancing food, exercise and insulin. It may, however, take quite a long time to find out the causes and from your question it is not clear whether all these factors have been looked at. Few patients have such difficulty in controlling their diabetes that they have to give up work. Was your doctor frightened that you might have a hypoglycaemic attack that would be hazardous in your particular job? If that was the case it might be better to look for a more suitable job rather than to rely on Social Security Benefits which are available to diabetics in the same way as they are to anyone else. There are some additional benefits available to the diabetic and for more details you should contact your local Social Worker at the diabetic clinic.

93 *I have noticed that there are much greater fluctuations in my blood sugar level when I am having a period. I have great difficulty in keeping blood sugar balanced then. I have read many books on diabetes but I have never seen this mentioned — is it normal?*

It is quite normal for the blood sugar control to fluctuate during the monthly cycle. Most patients find the blood sugar is highest in the pre-menstrual phase and returns to normal during or after the period. Some diabetics need to adjust their dose of insulin during the cycle but rarely by more than a few units. Every woman has to discover for herself the extent of this effect and how much extra insulin, if any, is needed. Your diabetic clinic doctor or specialist nurse is the best person to turn to for exact advice of how to make these adjustments.

94 *My daughter, who is 14 and has had diabetes for 3 years, is going through a difficult phase. In the past year she has had five admissions to hospital, one with a hypo and four with episodes of ketosis. From her attitude I suspect she is using her diabetes to manipulate us and probably also her teachers at school — is this a common occurrence? What should we do? We are desperately anxious not to upset her because she needs all the support we can give her. She does not find being a diabetic easy*

You have come across what I suspect is a very common problem and one that needs very careful handling.

Teenagers without diabetes can be fairly manipulative at times and it would be surprising if diabetic teenagers did not take advantage of their condition during this difficult phase in development. I am sure that you are quite right in putting love and devotion first in your list of priorities but closely behind that should be a gentle but firm attitude to discipline regarding the diabetes and attention to detail concerning regular monitoring and record keeping, regular injections and regular attendance for review. It is most important that your daughter should not get in the habit of missing insulin injections as this is the commonest cause of episodes of ketosis in this age group. It is particularly important to pay attention to the injection technique and the regularity of the injections. If you have any anxiety that she is deliberately missing these out then your best line is to insist on supervising them and her blood testing, etc., until she has demonstrated to you that she has matured enough to be able to keep things under control.

4

Life with diabetes

Introduction

This chapter is meant to answer all the questions that affect daily living when you are diabetic. It covers a broad sweep from sport and holidays to surgical operations and medical illness.

Some questions are trivial (e.g. 'Can I use a sunbed?'), and others are of great importance (e.g. 'Do I stop my insulin if I am sick?'). At the end of the chapter is a miscellaneous section with questions that we cannot find a place for (for example, Social Security Benefits, ear piercing and identity bracelets).

The section on other illnesses (p.161) should be read by all diabetics, so that they know how to react if they are struck down by a bad attack of flu. All car drivers should read the section on driving (p.167).

After reading this chapter, you should realize that there are few activities that are barred to diabetics. Provided that you understand the condition, you should be able to do almost anything you wish.

Sports

*1 My 13-year-old son is a keen footballer and has just been
diagnosed as diabetic. Will he be able to continue football
and other sports? If so, what precautions should he take?*

Your son can certainly keep on with his football. There are
several diabetics on insulin who play football for First
Division teams and for their country. If your son is good
enough at the game, diabetes should not stop him becoming
another great diabetic footballer. Diabetics have reached the
top in other sports, such as rugby, cricket, tennis, sailing,
orienteering and mountaineering. Certainly all normal
school sports should be encouraged. There is of course the
difficulty that the extra energy used on competitive sports
increases the risk of a hypo. Before any period of sport your
son should take some extra carbohydrate — sandwiches,
biscuits or chocolate wafer. Another snack at half-time is
usually necessary and he must carry glucose tablets in his
pocket.

Another way of preventing a hypo during exercise is to
reduce the amount of insulin beforehand. Thus if you are
playing football in the morning, you could reduce by half the
morning dose of quick-acting insulin. By trial and error you
will discover how much to cut your insulin for a given
amount of exercise.

A hypo during athletics and most team games can be
inconvenient and may reduce your son's dexterity, but a
hypo whilst swimming can be more serious. There are
certain rules all diabetics on insulin should follow before
swimming:

a Never swim alone.
b Tell your companions (or teacher) to pull you out of the
water if you behave oddly or are in difficulties.
c Keep glucose tablets on the side of the pool.
d Get out of the water immediately if you feel the first
signs of hypo.

By following these simple rules, diabetics can swim with
complete safety.

Unfortunately, diabetics on insulin are discouraged from scuba diving by the British Sub-Aqua Club.

2   *As a diabetic can I take part in all or any form of sport?*

The majority of sports are perfectly safe for diabetics. The problem lies in those sports where loss of control due to a hypo could be dangerous, not only to the diabetic but to fellow sportsmen or onlookers. Swimming is an example of a potentially dangerous sport but by taking certain precautions (see previous question) it is safe to swim. However, in other sports (e.g. scuba diving, motor racing) the risk of serious injury in the case of hypo are even greater. For this reason the governing bodies of these high-risk sports discourage diabetics from taking part.

3   *I understand that diabetics are banned from all forms of parachuting because of the risk of hypos. Surely if one was sensible and took extra carbohydrates before a jump the risk would be minimal as a jump only takes a few minutes. Please give your views on the subject*

I fully agree that it should be perfectly easy for a diabetic to ensure that he does not go hypo during the short time taken over a parachute jump. However, the British Parachute Association would be able to allow diabetics to jump only if their blood glucose were 7 mmol/l or more and that is probably why they have made the harsh decision of banning diabetics on insulin.

4   *As a 30-year-old insulin-dependent diabetic can I join a keep-fit class or do a work-out at home?*

Certainly. Keeping fit is important for everybody. If you are unused to exercise you should build up the exercises slowly each week so that you do not damage any muscles or tendons. Remember that exercise usually has the effect of lowering blood glucose so you may need to reduce your insulin dose or take extra carbohydrate before exercising. *The Diabetics' Get Fit Book* by Jacki Winter (published by Martin Dunitz) is an excellent, well-illustrated book that gives many suitable exercises for all ages and abilities.

5   *I am a diabetic on insulin and do quite a bit of jogging. I would like to try running a marathon. Have you any advice on the subject?*

Dr Matt Kiln, himself a diabetic on insulin, has considerable experience of long-distance running. He has passed on the following suggestions to other diabetics wishing to take up on this sport:

a   Wear comfortable clothes and proper running shoes. Watch out for blisters. Shorts should have a pocket for glucose sweets.

b   Start with short runs and build up slowly to longer distances. This should take 1½–2 years in young, fit people and even longer if you are older — perhaps as long as 4 years.

c   Aim at training three nights a week.

d   Regular running reduces the average daily insulin dose by about 25%. Once in training, you will probably need less insulin even on days that you are not running. Conversely more insulin will be needed once you get out of training.

e   During the run you will need to take carbohydrate. Glucose sweets are less likely to cause stomach cramps than Mars bars.

f   Measure blood sugar levels before and after each run and keep a careful record of the blood sugar values, distance, time taken, carbohydrate intake and time since last insulin injection. In this way you can build up a pattern of your likely glucose requirements for future runs.

g   On the day of a long run, if you reduce the insulin dose you will need to take less glucose while exercising. This lessens the risk of stomach cramps. Before the last London Marathon, Matt Kiln only gave himself 2 units of short-acting insulin. During the 41 km run (26.2 miles), which he achieved in 204 minutes, he only needed to take 30 g of carbohydrate (10 Dextrosol tablets). His blood sugar was 7 mmol/l at the start of the race and 4 mmol/l at the end. This perfect control was possible only because of careful measurements during the long training period.

h After the end of a long run the blood glucose tends to rise and you will probably need a small dose of insulin to counteract this.

Dr Kiln stresses that these hints are the result of his own personal experience and other diabetics may behave differently. Only 10% of the population as a whole is capable of finishing a Marathon. Nobody should run just for the glory. This activity should be (a) enjoyable and (b) help towards a better understanding and control of your diabetes.

Further advice is available from the BDA who will supply a copy of Dr Kiln's notes on the subject.

Eating out

6　*My wife and I entertain a great deal and we often go out to meals in a friend's house or in restaurants. I have recently been started on insulin for diabetes. How am I going to cope with eating out?*

It is sometimes difficult when eating out with friends who have made a special effort to prepare delicious food which is quite unsuitable for diabetics. Do you refuse a syrupy pudding and offend your hostess or have a large helping and to hell with your diabetes? It is probably less embarrassing to warn your hostess in advance that you are diabetic and have to avoid food containing high concentrations of sugar. Restaurants should be less of a problem as you can select from the menu dishes that are suitable.

People on two doses of insulin a day sometimes worry about how they are going to give their injections away from home. Nowadays with plastic syringes there should be no difficulty. You can retire to the lavatory just before sitting down to eat. Diabetics who are less shy can discreetly give themselves insulin into their abdomen or calf whilst at the table waiting for the first course to arrive. The use of the Penject (p.63) may also make the injection simpler as bottles of insulin do not need to be carried around. Do not take the evening dose of insulin before leaving home in case the meal is delayed.

Holidays/travel

*7   Do you have any simple rules for diabetics going abroad
for holidays?*

Here is a check-list:

a   Insulin.
b   Syringes.
c   Test strips (and finger pricker).
d   Identification bracelet/necklace/card.
e   Dextrosol tablets.
f   Glucagon.
g   Medical insurance.
h   Inside EEC — form E111 from the DHSS.

8   Is it safe for a diabetic to take travel sickness tablets?

Travel sickness pills do not upset diabetes though they may
make you sleepy so be careful how you drive. On the other
hand, vomiting can upset diabetes so it is worth trying to
avoid travel sickness. If you do become sick the usual rules
apply. Continue to take your normal dose of insulin and take
carbohydrate in some palatable liquid form (p.270). Test
blood or urine regularly.

*9   We are going on holiday and wish to take a supply of
insulin and glucagon with us. How should I store them
both for the journey and in the hotel?*

If travelling by air you should keep insulin in hand luggage as
temperatures in the luggage hold of an aircraft often fall
below freezing and insulin left in this luggage could be
damaged. Insulin is otherwise very stable and will keep for
months at room temperature in our temperate climate.
However, insulin can be damaged if kept too long at high
temperatures or if frozen. Insulin manufacturers say it is
stable for 1 month below 25°C (77°F), so it is perfectly safe
to keep insulin with your luggage on the average holiday.
Avoid the glove compartment or the boot of your car where
very high temperatures can be reached. In tropical
conditions your stock of insulin should be kept in the fridge.

It is best to carry your supplies in more than one piece of luggage in case one suitcase goes astray and you lose everything!

Storage of glucagon is no problem as this comes as a powder with a vial of water for dilution. It is stable and can survive extremes of heat and cold.

10 Many airports now X-ray baggage for security reasons. Does this affect insulin?

Fortunately not.

11 I would like to go on a skiing holiday. Is it safe for diabetics to ski, skate and toboggan? Should I take special precautions?

It is as safe for a diabetic to ski as it is for a non-diabetic. Accidents do occur and it is essential to take out adequate insurance to cover all medical expenses. Read carefully the small print in the insurance form to ensure that it does not exclude pre-existing diseases like diabetes, or require them to be declared. In this case you should contact the insurance company and if necessary take out extra medical cover for your diabetes. You should take all the usual precautions when travelling (see question 7). Physical activity increases the likelihood of hypos so always carry glucose and a snack as you may be delayed, especially if you are injured. Never go without a sensible companion who knows you are a diabetic and understands what to do if you have a hypo.

12 Is sunbathing all right for diabetics?

Of course diabetics can sunbathe. Lying around doing nothing may put your blood glucose up a bit — especially if you overeat, as most people do on holiday. So keep doing your usual tests, and you may need extra insulin; on the other hand, increasing the temperature of the skin may speed up the absorption of the insulin, so be prepared for changes.

13 Is vaccination more necessary in diabetics going abroad than non-diabetics?

Diabetics are no more or less likely to contract illnesses abroad than non-diabetics but if they do become ill the consequences could be more serious. Diabetics should have exactly the same vaccinations as anyone else. In addition to the necessary vaccinations it is very important to take protective tablets against malaria if you are going to a tropical area where this disease is found. More cases of this potentially serious disease are seen in this country, usually in travellers recently returned from Africa or the East.

14 I am going to work in the Middle East for 6 months. What can I do if my insulin is not available in the country where I am working?

If you are only working abroad for 6 months it should be quite easy to export with you enough insulin to last you this length of time. Kept in an ordinary fridge it should keep — but make sure you are not supplied with insulin which is near the end of its shelf life. The expiry date is printed on each box of insulin.

Most types of insulin are available in the Middle East but you may have to make do with a different brand name or even insulin from a different animal (pig, cow or human).

Strict Muslim countries regard pork and products from the pig as 'unclean' and porcine insulin may be hard to obtain in these countries. We have heard of customs officials in Saudi Arabia confiscating supplies of porcine insulin. To avoid this awkward situation it would be worth changing to beef or human insulin before you try to enter such a country. The change may affect your diabetic control; you should therefore make it in good time to allow yourself to stabilize before travelling. U 100 insulin may be difficult to obtain outside the UK, USA, Australia, New Zealand, South Africa and parts of the Far East. Most European countries only stock insulin in 40 u/ml, and special syringes for use with U 40 insulin will have to be obtained.

15 *My husband has just been offered an excellent post in Uruguay which he wishes to accept. He is worried about my diabetes there and especially about the availability of my insulin. Can you let me know if my insulin can be sent by post?*

It should be possible to obtain an equivalent type of insulin to your own in most parts of the world. If you are keen to keep up your normal supplies, Hypoguard Ltd are prepared to despatch syringes and equipment for testing blood and urine to all parts of the world. Unfortunately, Hypoguard are not able to handle insulin. You might be able to make arrangements with a high-street chemist who would be prepared to send insulin by post.

16 *My friends and I are going to Spain to work next year. One of my friends and I are diabetics. Can you tell me what I should take with me and whether I would have to pay if I needed to see a doctor?*

Before you go abroad prepare yourself well — take spares of everything such as syringes, insulin and testing equipment, and keep spare supplies separate from the main supply in case your luggage is lost. Do not leave insulin in the hold of an aircraft, where it might freeze.

Medical attention is free in all EEC countries although you should obtain certificate number E111 obtainable from your local Social Security office. For countries outside the EEC you should insure your health before you go. The Welfare Officer of the British Diabetic Association can help with this.

17 *I am a diabetic on insulin and need to fly to the USA. How do I cope with the changes in time zone?*

Flying from East to West (or vice versa) can be confusing at the best of times and makes it difficult to know which meal you are eating. Here are some typical schedules for travelling from London to the East and West Coasts of the USA plus the return trip.

1 London to New York
Get up as normal. Have usual dose of insulin and breakfast.

Departure 12.00 noon — have a good snack before boarding plane. Lunch and afternoon snack during flight.

Arrive 2.00 p.m. local time but your body thinks it is 7.00 p.m. Eat soon after arrival with your normal evening dose of insulin. If you then go to bed at 10.00 p.m. local time (3.00 in the morning to you) you will need a small dose of long-acting insulin before a well-earned sleep.

2 New York to London
The problem here is that most flights are in the evening and the night seems to be very short. Assuming that you are going to try to sleep on the plane, you should reduce your evening dose of insulin by one-third and have this at about 6.00 p.m. New York time followed by a reasonable meal. After take-off at 8.00 p.m. you should be served a meal and should then sleep. You will arrive at London at about 7.30 a.m. local time though it will feel to you like 2 a.m. Most people have another journey followed by a good meal and then a sleep. You should have a dose of long-acting insulin before this sleep and try to get back into phase by the evening (local time).

3 London to Los Angeles
This is an 11-hour flight, usually leaving around midday and arriving on the West Coast at 3.30 p.m. local time, which feels to you like 11.30 p.m. During this long flight you will have to have an injection of insulin on the plane and this is best if taken before dinner served at 6.00 p.m. London time. It would be safest to give half your normal evening dose as short-acting insulin and then try to sleep. On arrival at the other side you will need to travel to your destination and will probably have an evening meal which will feel to you like the early hours of the morning. A small dose of long-acting insulin before this meal would cover your subsequent sleep.

4 Los Angeles to London
Leave 6.30 p.m. and after a 10-hour flight you will arrive in London just after midday local time which will feel to you like 2.00 a.m. Meals on this flight are usually served about an hour after take-off and an hour before landing, in the hope that you have a good sleep between these two meals. One

way round this arrangement would be to have a dose of insulin immediately before the first meal, giving the normal dose of short-acting insulin and half the normal dose of long-acting insulin. Immediately before the second meal you could have a small dose of short-acting insulin alone. This should last you through until the normal evening meal at your destination which would be preceded by a routine evening insulin dose.

When travelling keep to the following rules:

a   Do not aim at perfect diabetic control. You have to be flexible especially on international flights. A hypo whilst travelling can be very inconvenient.
b   Be prepared to check your blood glucose if you are at all worried and not sure how much insulin you need.
c   In general, airlines are prepared to make special allowances for diabetics and air hostesses will do their best to help. Airlines say that they like to be warned in advance but in practice this should not be necessary.

Work

18   Can I undertake employment involving shift work?

Yes, certainly. Many diabetics combine shift work with control of their blood glucose. Shift work, however, does need a little extra care as most insulin regimens are designed round a 24-hour day. Shift workers usually complain that they are just settling into one routine when everything changes and they have to start again. It is hard to generalize about shift work as there are so many different patterns but if you follow these rules things should work out all right.

a   Aim at an injection of short- and medium-acting insulin every 12–16 hours.
b   Try to eat a good meal after each injection.
c   Eat your normal snacks between meals every 3 hours or so — unless you are asleep.

d   If there is a gap of 6–8 hours when you are changing from one shift to another, have some short-acting insulin on its own followed by a meal.

e   Because the pattern of insulin and food is constantly changing shift workers have to do more blood glucose measurements than normal as they cannot assume that one day is very much like another.

f   If the blood glucose results are not good be prepared to make changes in your dose of insulin. Soon you will know more about your diabetes than anyone else.

19   How can I cope with my diabetes if I work irregular hours as a sales representative?

Just as with shift work many diabetics manage to combine an irregular life-style with good diabetic control. Of course if you have had an injection of insulin in the morning and normally have a fairly low blood glucose before lunch, then you will go hypo unless you eat at the right time. So a well-controlled diabetic cannot afford the luxury of missing meals completely. However, it is always possible to have a few biscuits or even a sweet drink if you are getting past your normal time of eating. The occupational hazard of all sale reps, diabetic or otherwise, is the mileage they clock up each year on the roads. The dangers of hypoglycaemia while driving cannot be over-emphasized and there is really no excuse for this now that instant blood glucose measurement is available. Remember (1) if driving before a meal, check your blood glucose; (2) if it is low eat before driving; (3) carry food in your car and have some immediately if you feel warning of a hypo.

20   Should I warn fellow employees that I might be subject to 'hypos'?

Definitely. Hypos unfortunately do happen especially when a person first starts using insulin. Warn your workmates that if they find you acting in a peculiar way they must get you to take some sugar. Warn them also that you may not be co-operative at the time and may even resist their attempts to help you. Some people find it difficult to admit to their colleagues that they have diabetes. But if you keep it a secret you run the risk of causing a scare by having a bad hypo and being taken to hospital by ambulance for treatment. A needless trip to hospital should be avoided.

21 *My husband's hours of work can be very erratic. Sometimes he only gets 3 or 4 hours' sleep instead of his normal 8. Can you tell me what effect lack of sleep has on diabetes?*

Lack of sleep in itself will not affect diabetes though if your husband is under great pressure and the adrenaline is running very high, his blood glucose may be affected. The real problem with working under a strain is the tendency to ignore diabetes completely and assume that it will look after itself. Unfortunately a few minutes of each day has to be spent checking blood glucose, eating a snack or giving insulin. These minutes are well spent.

22 *Is it necessary for me to tell my friends and colleagues at work that I am diabetic?*

If you are on insulin, there is always the possible risk of hypoglycaemia, especially at the beginning when you are adjusting the dose of insulin and finding out about the effect of exertion on blood sugar. It is important to warn your workmates that if you behave in an odd way, they should give you some sugar. Show them where you keep your dextrose tablets.

If you are controlled on tablets, the risk of hypoglycaemia is very slight. However, you may well tell your workmates about your diabetes — it is nothing to be ashamed of.

23 *I became diabetic 5 months ago, 1 week after I had started a new job. I am coming to the end of my 6-month probation period and have been given 2 weeks' notice because of my diabetes. They said I could not do shift work because of my diabetes. Could you help?*

This is a sad story and a good example of ignorant prejudice against diabetics. Of course, there are many diabetics on shift work who maintain good control — though it does require a bit of extra thought. There is no way you can force your employer to keep you on, but you should ask your Clinic Doctor to get in touch with him, on your behalf. The BDA will also be prepared to write in your support.

24 *My daughter has recently been refused a place on a course for training in beauty therapy. Although nothing was mentioned in the cautiously worded refusal, I am convinced it is because of her diabetes. I would like your opinion on whether this profession is suitable for a well-controlled diabetic?*

A beauty therapist is a most suitable job for a diabetic. I know a girl who is in her second year of training as a beautician, and seems to be doing very well. She is at college at Nuneaton — perhaps your daughter should apply to join the same course.

25 *I am a Public House Manager and a diabetic for the past 19 years but my employers are now making me redundant. Apparently, their insurers cannot accept me for a permanent position owing to my diabetes. Who can help strengthen my case?*

I know of several publicans with diabetes who run good pubs and still keep their diabetes under good control. However, people who work in licensed premises do tend to drink more alcohol than average, and heavy drinkers are at great risk from hypos (p.171). I wonder if you have been having a large number of hypos which has made it difficult to continue in your present occupation. Ask your Clinic Doctor and the BDA to lobby on your behalf.

26 *I have been refused a job with a large company because of my diabetes. Have I sufficient grounds to take proceedings against them for discrimination?*

Unfortunately, there is no legislation to prevent prejudice against diabetics, so I do not think you would get anywhere by taking the company to court. We know that this sort of discrimination does sometimes happen, especially in large organizations, though, of course, it is very difficult to prove. It is hard to know how to overcome this sort of unspoken bias against diabetics.

It is the responsibility of diabetics who are at work to realize that they are, to some extent, on show. If they work well and have no time off for minor complaints, then the next diabetic who applies to the same firm will be looked on kindly and probably be taken on. On the other hand, someone who is constantly having hypos and missing work will give all diabetics a bad name.

The BDA has started to have meetings with Medical Officers responsible for the Occupational Health in large organizations, such as London Transport, the National Coal Board, British Rail and the Post Office. We hope that these will help to reduce prejudice over the next few years.

Other illnesses (colds, flu and depression)

27 *I have recently had a severe cough and cold and have been given medication suitable for diabetics by the doctor. Although I do not feel that my blood glucose is high, my urine tests have been 2% or more. Could this be due to the medication?*

This is a good example of the effect any infection or serious illness has on diabetes — it nearly always causes a rise in blood glucose. Unfortunately, diabetics often do not start to feel unwell until the glucose reaches danger level. Diabetics on insulin usually need more insulin when they are ill and yet they are sometimes advised to stop insulin completely if they do not feel like eating. This advice can be fatal. The rules when you are ill are:

a Test blood/urine frequently.
b If tests are high give extra doses of short-acting insulin.
c Never stop insulin.

It is of course possible to get over a bad cold by carrying on with your normal dose of insulin and accepting bad control for a few days. However, this means that your mouth and nose will be slightly dehydrated and it will take a few extra days before you feel back to normal. So you probably get better quicker if you adjust your insulin and try to keep the blood glucose near normal.

Antibiotic syrup and cough linctus are often blamed for making diabetes worse during an illness such as flu or chest infection. In fact a dose of antibiotic syrup only contains about 5 g of sugar and is not going to make any large difference. It is the illness itself that unbalances the diabetes. In general, medication from your doctor will not upset your diabetes. One antibiotic (Keflex) may cause a muddy colour of the urine which can be confusing.

28 *I have noticed that my son suffers from more colds since becoming diabetic. Could this be due to his diabetes?*

Many patients make this observation but there is no real reason why the common cold should be more common in diabetes. However, a relatively minor cold may upset the diabetic control and lead to several days of illness (see previous answer). This may make it a more memorable event. To repeat the previous advice, *never* stop insulin.

29 *My daughter keeps getting infections and has been rushed to hospital on several occasions with high ketones requiring a drip. How can I prevent these infections? Will vitamins help?*

It sounds as though your daughter is a so-called 'brittle' diabetic and this must be very alarming for you. There are two types of brittle diabetics. The first are those who are well controlled and can prove this by frequent blood glucose measurements below 7 mmol/l and a normal HbA_1 but who quickly become very ill and 'sugary' at the first sniff of a cold or the beginning of an infection. The other sort are those who are normally poorly controlled with variable blood glucose results and who therefore have no leeway when they become ill. In the case of the first type it should be possible to increase the dose of insulin rapidly giving extra doses every few hours depending on the blood glucose. The second type are more of a problem as it is the overall control which needs to be improved and this can be difficult (p.144). Of course if an identified infection (e.g. cystitis) starts off the trouble then this must be treated immediately with antibiotics.

Provided your daughter has a reasonable diet, vitamins will not help.

30 *My 6-year-old daughter who is insulin dependent is troubled with frequent vomiting which occurs suddenly. She has ended up in hospital on several occasions as she becomes dehydrated. What can I do to avoid this?*

Vomiting in a young diabetic child has to be taken seriously and the hospital admissions are probably necessary to put fluid back into your daughter by means of a drip. She sounds like another brittle diabetic and the previous answer applies. As she gets older these attacks of sickness will improve.

31 *What is the best treatment for a diabetic suffering from hay fever? I understand that some products can cause drowsiness which could affect my balance and so be confused with a hypo*

Diabetics may receive the same treatment for hay fever as non-diabetics as this does not affect diabetic control. Antihistamines are often used and these do make people feel sleepy but this should be easy to distinguish from a hypo. Remember that people on antihistamines should take alcohol with great caution. A long course of desensitizing injections can be tried but most hay-fever sufferers find this demands much time and effort for little reward. Hay fever can also be alleviated by sniffing capsules which reduce the sensitivity of the membranes in the nose.

32 *I have just been in hospital with anaphylactic shock from a bee sting. I am a diabetic controlled with tablets and wondered if this had anything to do with the severity of my reaction?*

There is no connection between diabetes and allergy to bees.

33 What is the effect of other illnesses on diabetes? Is my diabetic son likely to suffer more illness than other children of his age?

Illnesses usually make diabetes worse in the sense that people on insulin need to increase the dose to keep blood glucose controlled. Diabetics on tablets or diet alone often find that a bad cold will upset diabetic control. In the case of a prolonged illness or one needing hospital admission a 'mild' diabetic may need to have insulin injections for a time.

Diabetes itself does not necessarily make people prone to other illnesses. In fact a survey in a large American company reveals that diabetics had no more absences from work than non-diabetics. Most diabetic children grow up without any more illness than their non-diabetic friends.

34 Since I was diagnosed diabetic I have been very depressed. Is there any link between these two conditions?

People vary greatly in their mental response to becoming diabetic. Some lucky ones take to their new condition easily, while others, like yourself, find the whole thing very depressing. The depression seems to take two forms — firstly, shock and even anger at the very onset coupled with fear of injections and of the unspoken fear of complications. A few weeks later comes the depressing realization that diabetes is for life, and not just a temporary disease that can be 'cured'. This type of depression seems to affect young people who are presumably worried about their image and are feeling insecure about the future.

A few people with diabetes feel that, in some way, they are imperfect, especially if they have previously been fitness fanatics. The best way round this feeling of inadequacy is to throw yourself into sporting activities with extra enthusiasm. Exercise is good for us all and diabetics have managed to reach the top in most forms of sport from ocean-racing to international football.

If you treat your diabetes in a positive way rather than letting the condition control you, the depression will gradually lift.

35   *How does stress and worry affect diabetes? I spend*
     many hours studying and find that, if I study too long, I
     feel weak and my urine tests show negative. Are there
     any side-effects to pressure which may affect my
     diabetes?

In general, stress and worry tend to increase the blood
sugar. A Scottish student told me that in the run-up to her
final examination, she had to *double* her insulin dose to keep
perfect blood glucose control, even though she did not
appear to be particularly anxious to her friends. Stress
causes a release of adrenaline and other hormones which
antagonize the effect of insulin.

Also during periods of stress, it may be difficult to keep
strict meal times, so you could be going hypo. You need to
check your blood sugar and if it is not below normal, then you
are simply experiencing the tiredness we all feel after
studying hard. Do not blame it on your diabetes but have an
evening off from your studies.

Hospital operations

36   *Recently when I was in hospital to have my appendix*
     removed, I was put on a 'sliding scale'. Please could you
     explain this, especially as it might save other people in
     a similar position from worrying?

I agree that the expression 'sliding scale' does sound rather
alarming — but it is nothing to worry about. During and
after an operation it can be difficult to predict exactly how
much insulin a diabetic will need. The way round this is to
use a 'sliding scale' so that more insulin is given if the glucose
in the blood is high. In the past, a urine test would be done
every 4 hours and a certain dose of insulin would then be
given depending on the result of the test. Nowadays, during
an operation, insulin is often given straight into a vein using
a slow infusion pump. Many surgical wards have machines
for measuring blood glucose and by doing this every hour the
dose of insulin can be adjusted according to the result. In this
way, diabetic control can be carefully regulated throughout

the operation and until the patient is eating again. At this stage the insulin may be given by three injections a day, the dose given at each injection being determined from the blood glucose level according to the 'sliding scale'.

37 Are there any problems with surgery for the diabetic child?

Surgical operations with children usually entail a general anaesthetic and it is advisable to have nothing to eat or drink (nil by mouth) for 6 hours before the anaesthetic is given. Any difficulties caused by this period of fasting can be overcome by a glucose drip into the vein. The normal insulin injection is not given on the day of operation but small regular doses are either injected under the skin or pumped continuously into the vein. The dose of insulin is adjusted according to the blood glucose level.

In minor operations where the patient is expected to be eating an hour or so later, these elaborate procedures may not be necessary and insulin may simply be delayed until the next meal is due. If an emergency operation is necessary it is important that the doctors know that the patient is diabetic. This is another good reason for wearing an identification bracelet or necklace.

38 Must I tell my dentist I am a diabetic and will this affect my treatment in any way?

Being a diabetic will not affect your dentistry at all. However, it is important to remove all possibility of a hypo while in the dentist's chair. If you are on insulin, warn your dentist that you cannot run over a snack or meal time. It is less embarrassing to mention this before the start of a session than to have to eat dextrose while the dentist is trying to administer treatment.

Obviously, you must warn the dentist if he plans to give you any form of heavy sedation. If a diabetic on insulin is to have dentistry needing a general anaesthetic this is usually done in hospital.

39 Is a diabetic more likely to suffer from tooth decay or gum trouble?

There is an increased risk of infection in diabetics who are poorly controlled. The gums may become infected and this in turn may lead to tooth decay. However, a well-controlled diabetic is not prone to any particular dental problem — in fact, there is a positive advantage to avoiding sweets which cause dental caries.

Driving

40 I drive a lot in my work and lunchtime varies from day to day. Does this matter? I am on two injections of insulin a day

Yes, this can be a problem. The twice-daily insulin regimen is designed to provide a boost of insulin at midday to cope with the lunchtime intake of food. Once the early-morning injection of insulin has been given, there is no way of delaying the midday surge. It is common for people who are well controlled on two injections a day to feel a little 'hypo' before lunch.

There are three solutions to your problem:

1 Eat some biscuits or fruit while you are driving — only do this in emergencies as you will not know how much to have for lunch when you do get the chance to eat properly.

2 Change your insulin regimen so that you have a small dose of short-acting insulin before each main meal and only have long-acting insulin in the evening to keep your diabetes under control during the night. You would still have to eat snacks between meals but the three-injection method should make the timing of meals more flexible. With the new plastic syringes an extra injection is really no hardship.

3 Insulin pumps are not generally available to diabetics but they are likely to become more widely used in the future. The pump does free a diabetic from the inconvenience of fixed meal times.

41 *If I am taking insulin do I have to declare this in applying for a driving licence? If so am I likely to be required to furnish evidence as to fitness to drive?*

Anyone with diabetes whether needing insulin or not must declare this when applying for a driving licence. Once you have declared that you are diabetic, the DVLC (Driving and Vehicle Licencing Centre) will send you a form asking for details about your diabetes and the names of any doctors you see regularly. They also ask you to sign a declaration allowing your doctors to disclose medical details about your condition. There is usually no difficulty over a diabetic obtaining a licence to drive, though this will be valid for 3 years instead of up to the age of 70, which it is for most people in the UK. It is, of course, the risk of sudden and severe hypoglycaemia which makes diabetics liable to this form of discrimination. In general the only people who have difficulty in obtaining a 3-year licence are those on insulin with erratic control and a history of hypos causing unconsciousness. Once the condition has been controlled and severe hypos abolished, the diabetic may re-apply for a licence with confidence.

The following statement appears on every driving licence: 'You are required by law to inform the Drivers' Medical Branch DVLC Swansea at once if you have any disability (includes any physical or mental condition), which is or may become likely to affect your fitness as a driver, unless you do not expect it to last for more than 3 months'. This includes diabetes or any change in treatment from say, tablets to insulin. It is important to carry out these instructions as a diabetic who drives a car without informing the DVLC may find that his licence is invalid in the eyes of the law. Diabetics on insulin are not generally allowed to hold PSV or HGV licences.

42 *As a new diabetic I have had to have a form signed by my doctor for my insurance company to insure my car. The doctor charged me £2 for this service and pocketed the fee without even giving me a receipt. Is this normal?*

Motor insurance is another problem — in addition to the driving licence (p.168). Failure to inform your insurance company of your diabetes may make your cover invalid, in which case the consequences could be disastrous. The insurance company usually ask your doctor to complete a form. These forms vary but some of them are long and ask a lot of irritating and irrelevant questions. Unfortunately there is a charge of £2, but doctors are not obliged to sign these forms and are therefore entitled to a fee, just as you are entitled to a receipt. You may find that doctors at the hospital clinic will fill in the form for nothing.

Unfortunately there may be financial penalties for being a diabetic, and some insurance companies will load your premium. There is a wide variation from one company to another and it is worth shopping around for the 'best buy'. The British Diabetic Association can also help advise on insurance.

43 *I have heard that a diabetic driver who had a motor accident while 'hypo' was successfully prosecuted for driving under the influence of drugs and heavily fined. As a diabetic on insulin I was horrified to hear this verdict*

Several diabetics on insulin have been charged with this offence after a hypo at the wheel when the only 'drug' that they have used is insulin. It may seem unfair but for any victim of the accident, it is no compensation that the person responsible was hypo rather than being blind drunk. These cases emphasize the importance of taking driving seriously. Remember the rules:

a Always carry food/glucose in your car.
b If you feel at all hypo, stop your car and take some glucose.

c Preferably check that your blood sugar is above 5 mmol/l before driving again.

44 *I have been a bus driver for 15 years and was found to have diabetes 5 years ago. Until now I have been on tablets but may need to go on to insulin. Does this mean I will lose my job?*

As a bus driver you will hold a PSV (Public Service Vehicle) licence. Diabetics on insulin are not encouraged to hold a PSV. You are faced with a difficult choice — either to continue on tablets feeling unwell but holding down your job, or else to start insulin and feel much better, but risk losing your source of employment. I would have to advise you to go on to insulin as you will probably come to this eventually. Diabetics stabilized on insulin may hold a PSV unless their condition renders the driving of a PSV by them to be a likely source of danger to the public.

Any holder of a Heavy Goods Vehicle Licence (HGV) may also lose his licence and thus his livelihood if he has to start insulin treatment. He should be able to regain it once his treatment has stabilized. Diabetic HGV drivers who have already been on insulin for a number of years *may* be able to keep their licences provided they can prove that their diabetic control is good and they are not subject to hypos. The question of HGV licences is under review and at present a number of cases are going through the courts.

45 *I recently read a newspaper article which implied that diabetics who are breathalysed can produce a positive reading even though they have not been drinking alcohol. What does this mean?*

Diabetes has no effect on breathalyser tests for alcohol even if acetone is present on the breath. However, the new Lion Alcolmeter widely used by the police does also measure ketones, though this does not interfere with the alcohol measurement. Anyone breathalysed by the police may also be told that they have ketones and that they should consult their own doctor. These ketones may be caused either by diabetes which is out of control or by a long period of fasting.

Alcohol

*46   My husband likes a pint of beer in the evening. He has
      now been found to be a mild diabetic and has to stick to
      a diet. Does this mean he will have to give up drinking
      beer?*

No, he can still drink beer but if he is trying to lose weight he
will need to reduce his overall calorie intake and
unfortunately all alcohol contains calories. There are about
180 calories in a pint of beer, and this is equivalent to a large
bread roll. Special 'diabetic' lager contains less carbohydrate
but more alcohol so in the end it contains the same number of
calories, with the drawback of being more expensive and
more potent. So you husband is probably better off drinking
ordinary beer, but if he is overweight he will have to restrict
the amount he drinks (p.71).

*47   My teenage son has been diabetic since the age of 7. He
      is now beginning to show interest in going out with his
      friends in the evening. What advice can you give him
      about alcohol?*

Most diabetics drink alcohol and it is perfectly safe for them
to do so. However, if your son is on insulin he must be aware
of certain problems that alcohol can cause diabetics — in
particular alcohol can make hypos more serious. When
someone goes hypo a number of hormones are produced
which make the liver release glucose into the bloodstream. If
that person has drunk some alcohol, even as little as 2 pints
of beer, or a double gin, the liver will not be able to release
glucose and hypos will be more sudden and more severe. In
practice most alcoholic drinks also contain some carbohydrate which tends to *increase* the glucose in the blood. So
the overall effect of a particular alcoholic drink depends on
the proportions of alcohol to carbohydrate. For instance,
lemonade shandy (high carbohydrate/low alcohol) will have a
different effect on blood glucose from gin and Slimline tonic
(low carbohydrate/high alcohol). Your son may notice that
'diabetic' lager is more likely than ordinary beer to cause a
hypo because it contains less carbohydrate but more alcohol.

The best way for your son to discover how a certain alcoholic drink affects *him* is to do an experiment. He could stay at home one evening with a supply of his favourite drink and by measuring the blood glucose every hour would actually discover how different quantities of drink affected him. Someone else could also stay at home to do the blood tests for him. The experiment would provide useful information and could prevent an awkward experience later on. Diabetics are sometimes accused of being drunk when really they have become hypo after a modest amount of alcohol.

48 *I believe it is dangerous to drink alcohol when taking certain tablets. Does this apply to tablets used in diabetes?*

The answer is generally no. Some people on chlorpropamide (Diabenese) experience an odd flushing sensation when they drink alcohol but those patients can easily be changed to an equivalent tablet (e.g. glibenclamide) which does not cause this problem. The other consideration is that alcohol may alter someone's response to a hypo (see previous answer) and most tablets used for diabetes can cause hypos. If a patient on tablets is going to drink any alcohol he must be extra careful not to go hypo.

Drugs

49 *Is it true that diabetics taking vitamin C can get false results from Clinitest or Clinistix?*

Vitamin C is needed by the body in very small quantities and any excess is eliminated in the urine. Vitamin C may, in theory, react with Clinitest which is a test for reducing substances like glucose and vitamin C. In practice, people can take large amounts of vitamin C (up to 1 g a day) without affecting the Clinitest result. Clinistix is a specific test for glucose and will not be altered by vitamin C. The same applies to all blood testing strips.

50   Could the toxic effect of diazepam, Parstelin or Lentisol cause damage to the pancreas and, as a result, cause diabetes?

You mention examples from the three main groups of drugs used to treat depression and anxiety. None of these is known to have any affect on the pancreas or to be related in any way to diabetes.

51   My son was told that diabetics should not use Betnovate cream because it contains steroids. Is this true and why?

Most skin specialists avoid using powerful steroid creams such as Betnovate unless there is a serious skin condition. Often a weak steroid preparation or some bland ointment is just as effective in clearing up mild patches of eczema and other rashes. Unfortunately, the very strong steroids are often used first, instead of as a last resort. The strong steroids can be absorbed into the body through the skin and lead to a number of unwanted side-effects. This advice applies to all people with skin problems and not just diabetics. One of the side-effects of steroids is to cause a rise in the blood glucose level. Thus, a non-diabetic may develop diabetes while taking steroids and a diabetic treated with diet may need to go on tablets or insulin.

If there are good medical reasons for a diabetic to take steroids, in whatever form, he should be prepared to test his urine or blood for signs of poor control. If already taking insulin, the dose may need to be increased.

52   Can you tell me if any vaccination including BCG are dangerous in a diabetic?

There is no reason why a diabetic child should not have full immunization against the usual diseases. Sometimes the innoculation is followed by a mild flu-like illness which may lead to a slight upset of diabetic control. This is no reason to avoid protecting your child against measles, whooping cough and the rest. In some areas schoolchildren are given BCG as a protection against tuberculosis.

Diabetics should also have the normal immunization procedures if they are travelling to exotic places.

53 Is it harmful to take vitamin E and if not what is its value?

Vitamin E is important for maintaining potency in male rats. It has absolutely no effect on human beings. However, you may take this if it makes you feel better — it won't upset your diabetes.

54 I understand that aspirin lowers the blood sugar. Should I avoid taking it?

Large doses of aspirin given to diabetics not taking insulin may have a small effect in lowering blood glucose but in practice this does not cause any problem from hypoglycaemia. It has no effect on the blood glucose of insulin-treated patients. Aspirin can also cause indigestion and irritation of the stomach lining but this is not a particular risk for diabetics who may take aspirin and any other pain-killer in the same way as non-diabetics.

55 My wife suffers from severe indigestion. She is afraid to take indigestion tablets in case they upset her diabetes. Can you advise her what to do?

Indigestion tablets and medicines do not upset diabetes.

56 Is it safe to take diuretics ('water tablets') if one is diabetic?

Diuretics are given to people who are retaining too much fluid in their body. This may happen in heart failure and cause swelling of the ankles or shortness of breath. Diuretics are usually effective but, as a side-effect, they may cause a slight increase in the blood glucose. This is especially true of the milder diuretics such as Navidrex, which belong to the thiazide group. The increase in sugar is only slight but can sometimes mean that a patient controlled on diet alone may need to take tablets. Diabetics already on insulin are not affected by diuretics. The thiazide group of tablets is also used in the treatment of raised blood pressure.

57 Can you tell me if hormone replacement therapy is suitable for diabetics?

Hormone replacement therapy is given to women who are suffering unpleasant symptoms, usually 'hot flushes' around the time of the menopause. Hormone replacement therapy is not usually given to people with certain conditions such as strokes, thrombosis, high blood pressure, liver disease or gallstones. This treatment may have a slight worsening effect on diabetes similar to the pill (p.191 and p.195). Some doctors are reluctant to use these hormones in any patient and may use diabetes as an excuse for not prescribing them. However, small doses of female hormones can cause dramatic relief of severe menopausal symptoms and there is no reason why diabetics should not benefit from them provided there is no history of strokes, thrombosis, etc.

58 Is there any special cough mixture for diabetics?

Yes. Various sugar-free cough mixtures (e.g. Dia-Tuss) which can be prescribed by your doctor. However, there are only a few grams of sugar in a dose of ordinary cough mixture and this amount is not going to have an appreciable effect on the level of blood glucose. So you can give ordinary cough mixtures in moderate amounts to a diabetic child.

59 I have been on insulin for diabetes for 7 years. I was recently found to have raised blood pressure and was given tablets, called beta-blockers, by my doctor. Since then I have had a bad hypo in which I collapsed without the normal warning signs of sweating, shaking, etc. Could the blood pressure tablets have caused this severe hypo?

Beta-blockers are widely used for the treatment of high blood pressure and certain heart conditions. They have an 'anti-adrenaline' effect which sometimes damps down the normal 'adrenaline' response to a hypo (p.34). Thus, the low blood sugar may prevent someone thinking clearly without the normal sweating and shaking that warns of an impending hypo. Some beta-blockers have been designed to have their effect only in the heart without blocking the general adrenaline reaction of the body. These are theoretically much safer for diabetics taking insulin.

If you are already taking beta-blockers and having no unexpected problems from hypos, then you should carry on without worry. If you are taking beta-blockers for the first time, you should be warned by your doctor that your reaction to a hypo may be blunted. If this problem does occur, your doctor should either try a different beta-blocker or some other type of treatment for blood pressure.

60   Please could you give me a list of tablets or medicines which may interfere with my diabetes?

The important medicines which affect diabetics have been dealt with in this section. There are no medicines which must never be used but the following *may* increase the blood glucose and upset diabetic control:

a   Steroids (e.g. prednisolone, Betnovate ointment). Steroid inhalers (e.g. Becotide) should not have any ill effect.
b   Thiazide diuretics (e.g. Navidrex, Neo-Naclex).
c   The contraceptive pill.
d   Hormone replacement therapy (e.g. Harmogen, Progynova).
e   Certain bronchodilators (e.g. Ventolin) may have a slight effect on raising the blood glucose.

Aspirin in large doses may lower blood glucose.
Beta-blockers (e.g. Inderal, Tenormin) may prevent diabetics on insulin from recognizing a hypo (p.34).

Smoking

61 *I am a 16-year-old diabetic on insulin. I would like to know whether smoking low-tar cigarettes could interfere with my diabetes? Would it cause any restriction in my diet?*

Smoking is unhealthy not only because it causes cancer of the lung but because it leads to hardening of the arteries — affecting chiefly the heart, brain and legs. The proper advice to all diabetics, especially teenagers, is *not* to smoke. Smoking will not directly affect diabetic control except, perhaps, by reducing your appetite.

62 *When my doctor diagnosed diabetes, he told me to stop smoking. Could you tell me if there is a particular health hazard associated with smoking as a diabetic? The problem is made worse for me by the fact that I have to lose weight and if I stop smoking I will do just the opposite*

Smoking is a danger, not only to the lungs but because of the risk of increased arterial disease affecting any smoker. The long-standing diabetic is also at risk of problems with poor blood circulation. It is foolish to double the diabetic risk by continuing to smoke. If the discovery that you are diabetic has come as an unpleasant surprise, this is a good time to turn over a new leaf and alter your life-style — by eating less and giving up cigarettes. It may be a lot to ask, but many people manage to carry out a 'double' — it will not kill you. On the contrary, you may live longer.

63 *Since my husband, who has been diabetic for 23 years, has stopped smoking, he has not had a negative urine test. Why?*

Your husband should be congratulated for giving up smoking. Presumably he has been smoking for even more than 23 years. Most people who give up smoking do put on weight, on average 4 kg (9 lb). Presumably, this is because cigarettes suppress the appetite and people feel the need of another form of oral gratification when they stop smoking. If your husband has put on weight, this explains why his diabetes has gone out of control. If so, then he must reduce weight and his diabetes should improve. If he is already thin and his blood sugars are high then he will have to take tablets or insulin to get things under control.

Miscellaneous

64 Is there any objection to my donating blood? I am on two injections of soluble insulin a day and my general health is fine

There is no obvious reason why a fit diabetic should not be a blood donor. However, the blood transfusion authorities do not accept blood from a diabetic on insulin. They suggest that the antibodies to insulin found in all diabetics having injections may in some mysterious way harm the recipient of the blood. The transfusion service, however, welcomes donors who are diabetics but not on insulin.

65 My mother has been diabetic for 12 years and is subject to crashing hypos for no reason. She needs someone to be with her all the time. Would we be eligible for an Attendance Allowance as she needs watching 24 hours a day?

If you have to provide a continuous watch over your mother then you would be able to apply for an Attendance Allowance. Before admitting defeat, however, it would be better to try every means to prevent the hypos. Presumably your mother is having insulin, though you do not mention the dose or type of insulin she takes. At a guess, she is having a large dose of Lente insulin every morning. This method of giving insulin sometimes leads to severe hypos at unexpected times of the day or night. Changing to more frequent but smaller doses of insulin might solve the problem. You may have to spend a lot of time and energy to control your mother's diabetes. It would do more for her self-confidence to abolish the hypos than to get an Attendance Allowance.

66   *Since becoming diabetic I have found that my food bills
     have risen alarmingly. Are there are special allowances
     I can claim to offset the very high cost of the food?*

Most diabetics are not entitled to any special allowance and,
indeed, there is no real need for them to eat different food
from others. Special 'diabetic' products are not necessary
and if eaten at all should be treated as luxuries. Now that
diabetics are encouraged to eat food that is high rather than
low in carbohydrate, they do not have to fall back on
expensive protein as a source of calories.

Diabetics who are on Supplementary Benefit or those with
low incomes may be entitled to a discretionary diet
allowance by Social Security. In July 1984 the maximum was
£1.45 per week.

Students receiving a grant may also be eligible for a
supplementary allowance if they are a diabetic on insulin.

67   *To what Social Security benefits am I entitled now that
     I am diabetic?*

There are no special benefits given automatically to
diabetics. Those on supplementary benefit may apply for a
diet allowance (see previous question). However, there
should not be any additional cost attached to diabetes. At
present people using plastic syringes have to pay for them,
but they should not cost more than 25p per week. Insulin or
tablets will be provided on prescription and all diabetics do
have the one financial advantage of being exempt from *all*
prescription charges.

68   *I have just learnt that our son is a diabetic and I wonder
     if there is a special income tax allowance available?*

No. Sorry.

69   *My local youth group is holding a sponsored fast over a
     weekend. I am an insulin-requiring diabetic — can I
     take part?*

It would be difficult and perhaps dangerous for you to go
without food and, even more important, drink for 48 hours.

The problem is that even in the fasting state you need small amounts of insulin to prevent the blood sugar rising. Having taken insulin, you would then need food to prevent an overshoot leading to a hypo. Anyone who goes without food for long periods produces ketones and these could be an additional hazard in a diabetic.

70 *Is it true that a diabetic should not use an electric blanket?*

It is perfectly safe for a diabetic to use an electric blanket though underblankets should only be used to warm up the bed in advance. The manufacturers recommend that underblankets should be switched off before getting into bed — tempting though it is to lie on one warming yourself.

Hot-water bottles are rather more dangerous as the temperature is not controlled. Diabetics with a slight degree of nerve damage can fail to realize that a bottle full of very hot water may be burning the skin of their feet. This is a common cause of foot ulcers in diabetics. It is better to be safe than sorry and avoid the comfort of a hot water bottle.

71 *My daughter is 10 and has had diabetes for 3 months. She has started to lose a lot of hair and now has a bald patch. Is this connected with her diabetes?*

Yes, it could be. There are three ways in which diabetes and hair loss may be connected:

a   If your child was very ill with ketoacidosis at the time of the diagnosis, this could lead to a heavy loss of hair. If this is the case, the hair will re-grow over the next few months.

b   Alopecia areata is a skin condition which is *slightly* more common in diabetes. This is the likely diagnosis if your daughter has a well-defined bald patch with the rest of the hair remaining a normal thickness. If the patch is on the top of the head there is every chance that the hair will re-grow over the next 6 months. There is no way of encouraging growth and steroid ointments may even cause permanent skin changes and make matters worse.

c Myxoedema or lack of thyroid hormones may occur with diabetes. If this is the cause of your daughter's hair loss you will notice other symptoms such as mental slowing, weight increase and an inability to keep warm. All these symptoms can be corrected by taking thyroid tablets.

Shortage of body iron may also cause hair loss though this is not connected with diabetes.

72 *My hair is thinning all over and my doctor tells me that it is because of the Isophane insulin I am taking. Please could you tell me whether insulin affects hair growth?*

Baldness is not caused by Isophane insulin — or any other insulin for that matter. See previous question for the relationship between hair and diabetes.

73 *I recently enquired about having electrolysis treatment for excess hair. I was told that, as a diabetic, I would need a letter from my doctor stating that my diabetes did not encourage hair growth. Could I use wax hair removers instead?*

There is no objection to diabetics having electrolysis. Diabetes does not cause excessive hair growth. It sounds as though the firm doing the electrolysis are keen to turn away customers.

Many women find wax hair removers useful for the less sensitive parts of the body. Make sure that it is not too hot.

74 *Is it safe for diabetics to use sunbeds and saunas?*

As safe as for non-diabetics. Exposure to ultraviolet radiation is known to increase the risk of skin cancer.

Make sure you can recognize a hypo when you are hot and sweaty. Keep some means of treating a hypo with you — not with your clothes in the changing room.

75 *Can I wear contact lenses and if so would you recommend the hard or soft ones?*

Diabetes should not prevent the use of contact lenses or influence the type of lens you are given. You must have them prescribed by a qualified optician and it would be sensible to let him know that you are diabetic. Like anyone else with contact lenses, you will have to be careful to avoid eye infections.

76 *I would dearly love to have my ears pierced but when I asked my doctor about this, he said there was a chance that my ears would swell. Please could you advise me if there is a great risk of this happening?*

Anyone who has their ears pierced runs a small risk of infection until the wound heals completely. The risk in a well-controlled diabetic is no higher than normal. If the ear does become red, swollen and painful, you will need an antibiotic.

77 *Is there any connection between vertigo and diabetes? I have been diabetic for 2½ years controlled on a diet alone*

Vertigo in the strict medical sense describes that awful feeling when the whole world seems to be spinning round. It is usually due to disease of the inner ear or the part of the brain that controls balance. This is not connected with diabetes in any way. However, simple dizzy spells are a common problem with many possible causes which may be difficult to diagnose. If dizziness occurs when you move from sitting down to the standing position, it may be the result of a sudden fall in blood pressure. This can sometimes be due to a loss of reflexes from diabetic neuropathy (p.246). There are no other connections between diabetes and 'vertigo'.

78 *My husband's grandmother is 84 and a diabetic. Although she is fiercely independent, she cannot look after herself properly and will have to go into a home. Can you let me know of any homes which cater especially for diabetics?*

Because diabetes becomes increasingly common in the elderly, most old people's homes are well experienced in looking after diabetics. The staff of the home will probably be happy to do urine tests, ensure that diet is satisfactory and give the old lady her tablets and, if necessary, insulin injections. If your grandmother-in-law is too fit and independent to accept an old people's home, she may be a suitable candidate for a warden-controlled flat.

79 *My wife, who was diagnosed diabetic a few weeks ago, is about to return to work. I feel that she should wear some sort of identify disc or bracelet showing she is diabetic but she is relunctant to wear anything too eye-catching. Have you any suggestions?*

It is important that all diabetics, especially those on insulin, should wear some form of identification. Accidents can and do happen and it may be vital that any medical emergency team knows that your wife is diabetic.

Medic-Alert (11/12 Clifton Terrace, London N4 3JP) provide alloy bracelets or necklets which are functional if not very beautiful.

SOS/Talisman, Golden Key Co. Ltd, 9–11 High Street, Sheerness, Kent, produce a medallion which can be unscrewed to reveal identification and medical details. These can be bought in most jewellers and come in a wide range of styles and prices, including those in 9-carat gold.

Alternatively, your wife might prefer a do-it-yourself disc or bracelet inscribed, *DIABETIC ON INSULIN*. This could be effective without being too 'eye-catching'.

80 *Could you tell me what ointment to use for diabetic skin irritation?*

The most common cause of skin irritation in diabetics is itching around the genital region (pruritis vulvae). The most important treatment is to eliminate glucose from the urine by controlling diabetes. However, the itching can be relieved temporarily by cream containing a fungicide (e.g. nystatin).

81 *I believe that diabetics are entitled to free prescriptions. Please could you tell me how to apply?*

One of the few definite advantages of being diabetic is exemption from payment on all prescription charges — even for treatment which is not connected to the diabetes itself.

You must obtain a form entitled *NHS Prescriptions — How to Get Them Free* (Form C-P11/82) from a chemist, hospital pharmacy or a Post Office. Having filled in the form yourself, it must be signed by your family doctor or clinic doctor and sent to the local Family Practitioner Committee. The chemist should be able to give you the address. You will, in due course, receive an exemption certificate. Please remember to carry this certificate wherever you are likely to need a prescription, for instance when going to the diabetic clinic or going on holiday in the UK.

5

Sex and contraception

Introduction

Although modern society has removed many of the taboos
and inhibitions about sex and contraception, many people
still find it a difficult subject to ask personal questions about.
There are very many old wives tales about diabetes and sex
and most of these are rubbish. Basically, diabetics are no
different from non-diabetics in any aspect of sex, sexuality,
fertility, infertility and contraception. There are, however, a
few exceptions such as the undoubted risk of impotence in
long-standing male diabetics with evidence of extensive
neuropathy. Even this has to be considered in relationship to
the fact that impotence is a very common problem in non-
diabetics and there is no good evidence to show that
diabetics do in fact have more problems than a carefully
matched group of non-diabetics. There is certainly good
evidence that the female diabetic is totally without risk of
developing any problem analogous to impotence. Frigidity,
on the other hand, is common in both diabetic and non-
diabetic women just as impotence is common in diabetic and
non-diabetic men.

Various contraceptive devices have at times been claimed
to be less effective in diabetics — the evidence to support
this is poor and in our opinion diabetics should consider

themselves entirely normal as far as contraceptive practice is concerned.

There was, in the 1960s and 1970s, much emphasis on the potential risk of precipitating diabetes in non-diabetics taking oral contraceptives. It is now felt that the risks were grossly exaggerated in the press.

Impotence

1 Does diabetes affect the sex life (especially in males)?

No. The vast majority of diabetics, both male and female, are able to lead a completely full and normal sex life. This does not mean that problems do not occur but that the vast majority of these problems have nothing to do with diabetes. If, for any reason, diabetic control is lost with severe hyperglycaemia then this can affect sex life. In a minority of long-standing diabetics who have either bad neuropathy or arterial disease a loss of sexual potency can be directly attributed to diabetes but this is extremely uncommon and the majority of diabetics, both male and female, can look forward to a completely normal sexual life.

2 Is it normal for a diabetic to suddenly find themselves totally disinterested in sexual intercourse?

No more so than in non-diabetics. The feeling you describe is more common in females than in males but no more common in diabetics than in non-diabetics.

3 Does a low blood sugar affect the ability to achieve or maintain an erection and more importantly, the ability to ejaculate?

No, unless the blood sugar is very low (less than 2 mmol/l) when it is possible to show that many aspects of neurological function are transiently impaired and this can effect both potency and ejaculation.

4   *Is there some drug or hormone which will help cure impotence?*

It is extremely rare for impotence to be due to a hormonal abnormality. The majority of cases of impotence are due to psychological causes and often respond to appropriate advice and occasionally to drug treatment. If there is a hormonal defect, hormone replacement treatment will cure that particular form of impotence. It is essential to get a correct diagnosis to ensure appropriate therapy.

5   *I am a man of 43 years and have been a diabetic for 33 years. I intend to get married in the near future but I find that over the past 5 years my sex life lets me down when I am with the opposite sex. When I am on my own I am all right apart from my staying power. The hospital could find nothing wrong and thought it may be due to my diabetes — is there anything that can be done to help me?*

It sounds as if your problems are psychological rather than physical. If your diabetes is well controlled and the hospital can find no evidence of neuropathy, then the best advice is to proceed with your marriage but discuss the problem fully with your fiancée. She will then give sympathy and help to overcome what we are sure will be only a temporary problem.

6   *This impotency quietly worries me, it must be causing many diabetics similar worries*

From your question we understand that it is the possibility of your becoming inpotent that causes you most worry. Many diabetics undoubtedly worry about possible complications which may lay ahead of them, and all male diabetics have loss of potency at the top of their worry list. Our advice to you is worry more about keeping your diabetes under control and balanced and less about what skeletons there could be in the cupboard. By ensuring that you have good diabetic control you are doing everything that you possibly can to avoid trouble in the future and the chances are that you will steer clear of trouble throughout your life.

7 *My wife left me because I was impotent and the doctors say that there is nothing they can do for me — why was I not told about this?*

Are you sure impotence is the only reason why your wife left? I am surprised that the doctors said that there is nothing they can do for you, because even for those who are completely impotent there are surgical implants which have been successful in many cases. No doubt you feel aggrieved and would like to find someone to blame for the breakdown of your marriage. It sounds as if your impotence became a flashpoint for domestic rows. In my experience, most wives are sympathetic and understanding about impotence (whatever the cause) provided both partners can talk about the matter in an open manner. I have known a frank discussion lead to an increase of affection within marriage. Keeping things bottled up leads to the aggression and resentment that emerges from your question.

8 *I have had trouble keeping an erection for the last few months — has this anything to do with my diabetes? I also had a vasectomy a few years ago*

This is a difficult question to be able to answer without knowing more about your medical history. Certainly it is unlikely that the vasectomy has anything to do with your current problem. Failure to maintain an adequate erection may occasionally be an early symptom of diabetic neuropathy. However, at least as commonly, it is a symptom of growing older and we would need to do detailed tests on you to be quite sure what exactly is the cause.

9 *My fiancé suffers from impotence, and is attending a psychiatrist specializing in sexual problems. The psychiatrist says that his impotence has nothing to do with his diabetes but I have read that diabetics are prone to this*

Undoubtedly the commonest cause of impotence in diabetics is psychological problems of one sort or another, and though diabetic neuropathy can cause impotence, it is not usually the cause.

10   *I suffered a stroke affecting the right side of my body 12 months ago at the age of 40 and now suffer from partial impotence. The onset seemed to coincide not with the stroke but with taking anticoagulants. Are these known to cause impotence? I have heard that blood pressure tablets can cause impotence. I have been taking these for 3 months and wonder whether this is a factor?*

A severe stroke can sometimes be associated with impotence. A stroke is often due to narrowing of the arteries inside the head; the arteries elsewhere may also be narrowed and if the ones supplying blood to the genital organs are affected then it could contribute to your impotence. You are also quite right about the question of drugs. Some blood pressure lowering drugs may cause impotence and can interfere with ejaculation. It is sometimes possible to change to alternative drugs but there is no certainty that this will help the problem. It would be unwise to stop taking the drugs since this would lead to loss of control of your blood pressure. I suggest you consult your doctor and ask him if he is prepared to try an alternative from of tablet treatment for your high blood pressure.

11   *My husband, who is a middle-aged insulin-dependent diabetic, has been impotent for the past 2 years. Please will you explain his condition as I am worried that my teenage son, who is also diabetic, may also discover that he is impotent. It is difficult to discuss this with the doctor as he is unsympathetic*

I am sorry that you find it is difficult to discuss this with your own doctor. This is a subject some people find embarrassing but it is an important question that is always being raised by diabetics. Impotence (or the fear of it) worries and upsets many people; it is certainly not so rare that we can ignore it. It has been claimed that as many as 20% of diabetic men (though the figure is probably not as high as this) may at some stage become impotent. Most impotent men are not suffering from diabetes: anxiety, overwork, tiredness, stress, guilt, alcohol excess and grief can cause or contribute to impotence. It is not uncommon for any man to find at some stage that he is temporarily impotent and there is no reason why diabetic men should not also experience this. Anxiety that this failure induces can perpetuate the condition. Overwork or worry is frequently the cause of lack of interest in sex and even of impotence. Excess alcohol can cause prolonged lack of potency.

Some diabetics do become impotent, usually due to an impairment of the nerve supplying the penis. This usually takes time to develop and in the younger insulin-dependent diabetic we believe it can be prevented by strict blood sugar control. In the older patient (whose diabetes may appear to be 'milder') the condition responds less readily to treatment probably because the blood sugar has been high for a long time before the diabetes was diagnosed. In this age impotence is more commonly due to other factors and not diabetes. I hope you will be encouraged to discuss the matter further with your own doctor or with the doctor in the diabetic clinic where your husband and son attend.

12   *I have recently become impotent at the age of 30. My doctor tells me that this is not due to my diabetes. However, I am inclined to believe that being diabetic must be a contributory factor. Can you tell me if there is any connection between diabetes and impotence?*

There are, as you may know, many causes of impotence. It can occur with any severe illness but psychological causes are probably the commonest whilst diabetes is less frequently at fault. When impotence occurs in diabetes it may be due to diabetic neuropathy (nerve damage) which sometimes affects older diabetics with diabetes of many years duration, this would be a very unusual occurrence at 30 years of age. Where the cause of the impotence is reversible (for example after recovery from severe illness of whatever kind, or with recovery from depressive illness) then the impotence also recovers. It is difficult sometimes to decide if impotence is the result of diabetic neuropathy but when it is, recovery is unusual. Of course there are plenty of diabetics with neuropathy who are not impotent; this may seem rather confusing but diagnosis of the cause of impotence is rarely easy and specialist counselling and examination may be needed. There are many centres which offer counselling for those suffering from impotence, the facilities which are available vary from one part of the country to another and it is best to take the advice of your general practitioner or your diabetic clinic who will know the best local arrangement.

13 After sexual intercourse I recently suffered quite a bad hypo. Is this likely to happen again and if so, what can be done to prevent it?

This form of physical activity can, like any other, lower the blood sugar level of insulin-treated diabetics and lead to hypoglycaemia. When this happens — it is not uncommon — then the usual remedies need to be taken: more food or sugar beforehand or immediately afterwards.

The pill, IUD and vasectomy

14 Are there any extra risks that diabetic women run in using the contraceptive pill?

Use of the oral contraceptive pill carries the same risks in diabetics and in non-diabetics alike. It is now well known that the pill carries with it small risks — although these are obviously less than the risks of pregnancy itself. This is why all women are examined and questioned before starting the pill because there are a few conditions in which it is best avoided and other methods of contraception used. The same arguments apply equally to diabetics and non-diabetics. Healthy diabetic women who have been checked the same way as non-diabetics may certainly use the pill and there are no additional risks. When diabetics start using the pill there is sometimes a slight deterioration of control, this is rarely a problem and usually easily dealt with by a small increase of treatment which in those taking insulin may mean a small increase in insulin dose. It is a simple matter to monitor the blood or urine level and make appropriate adjustments.

There is nothing to suggest that the pill causes diabetes when taken by non-diabetics. It is all right for the non-diabetic relatives of diabetics to use the pill but of course they, like others, should attend for regular checks by their general practitioner or Family Planning Association.

15 *Is the contraceptive pill safe for insulin-dependent diabetics?*

Yes.

16 *I have just started the menopause and wondered if diabetics have to wait 2 years after the last period before doing away with contraception?*

Although the periods may become irregular and infrequent at the start of the menopause it is still possible to be fertile and this advice is precaution against unwanted pregnancy and applies equally to diabetics and non-diabetics.

17 *My doctor prescribed the pill for me but on the packet it states that they are unsuitable for diabetics. As my doctor knows that I am a diabetic is it safe enough for me?*

Yes. There used to be some confusion about whether the pill was suitable for diabetics but this has been resolved and there is general agreement that diabetics may use the pill for contraceptive purposes without any increased risks compared with non-diabetics.

18 *I am a diabetic and I am marrying another diabetic in 8 weeks' time. Please could you advise me on how to stop becoming pregnant?*

I am not quite clear from your letter whether you wish to be sterilized and not have children or whether you are just seeking contraceptive advice. If you and your fiancé have decided that you do not want to have the anxiety of your children inheriting diabetes and you have made a clear decision not to have children, then you have the option of your fiancé having a vasectomy or yourself being sterilized.

These are both fundamental decisions and will require careful thought because they are probably best considered as irreversible procedures. But if you are quite clear in this plan then they are probably the best procedures to consider. My advice would be to discuss this jointly with your GP and seek referral either to a surgeon for vasectomy for your fiancé or to a gynaecologist for sterilization. Whichever referral you get, it will be important for both of you to attend since no surgeon is going to undertake this procedure unless he is absolutely clear that you have thought about it carefully and have come to a clear, informed decision. If my interpretation of your question has not been right and you are merely looking for contraceptive advice then the best source of this is either your GP or the local Family Planning Clinic.

19 *Can you please give me any information regarding vasectomy and any side-effects it may have for diabetics?*

Vasectomy is a relatively minor surgical procedure which comprises cutting and tying off the vas deferens which is the tube that conveys the sperm from the testicle to the penis. Vasectomy may be carried out under either local or general anaesthesia, usually but not always as a day case. As a diabetic you may be advised that it would be simpler to have it under local anaesthesia since in this way your eating should not be affected and the balance of your diabetes not disturbed. The side-effects of the operation are primarily discomfort although infections and complications do rarely occur. The only special effects it would have on you as a diabetic are related to any disturbance that may occur in your balance as a result of having to go into hospital or having to have an anaesthetic.

There are a few medical reasons for avoiding this operation but they apply equally to non-diabetics as they do to diabetics.

20 *Is the 'progesterone only' pill suitable for diabetics?*

Yes, although recently these have become less popular both for diabetics and non-diabetics.

21 *I have been warned that IUDs (Intra Uterine Contraceptive Devices) are more unreliable in diabetics than non-diabetics, is this really true?*

IUDs are generally regarded as slightly less reliable contraceptives than the pill and there has been one report suggesting they may be even less reliable when used by diabetics. Not all experts agree about this, since there are no other reports containing this observation. There has also been a report suggesting that diabetics may be slightly more susceptible to pelvic infections when using the IUD. On balance, our recommendation is that IUDs should be considered as effective and useful in diabetics as in non-diabetics.

Thrush

22 *I keep getting recurrence of vaginal thrush and my doctor says that as a diabetic there is nothing that I can do about this — is this correct?*

Thrush is due to an infection with a yeast that thrives in the presence of sugar. If your diabetes is badly controlled and you are passing large amounts of sugar in the urine then you will be susceptible to thrush and however much ointment and cream you use it is likely to recur. The best line of treatment is to control your diabetes so well that there is no sugar in the urine and then the thrush will disappear probably without the need for any antibiotics, although antibiotics will speed the healing process. As long as you keep your urine free from sugar you should be free from any recurrence of the thrush.

23 *I am a diabetic with thrush. I have been well controlled*
for 10 years now. I do regular blood tests and most of
them are less than 10 mmol/l and when ever I check a
urine test it is always negative. I have been taking the
oral contraceptive pill for 3 years and I understand both
diabetes and the pill predispose one to thrush — can
you advise me what to do?

Since your diabetes is well controlled and your urine
consistently free from sugar diabetes can probably be
excluded as a cause of the thrush. One has to presume that in
your case it is a relatively rare side-effect of the pill, and you
would be best advised to seek alternative forms of
contraception.

Hormone replacement therapy

24 *During the past 5 years I have had trouble with my*
periods being very heavy and on several occasions I
have become very anaemic. I have tried hormone
replacement therapy (HRT) which interferes with my
diabetic control and it has been suggested that I have a
hysterectomy. I have heard that depression is common
after this operation and that HRT is often given to
alleviate this feeling but if this treatment makes
diabetic control more difficult, how will I cope? I realize
that I should ask both my diabetic and gynaecological
consultants these questions but I never seem to ask the
right questions when being interviewed

Many . people do have the impression that following
hysterectomy depression is common. There is no reason for
this. Anyone might get a little bit depressed after an
operation in the same way as he or she would after an illness.
A few women may feel that if they have their womb removed
they have lost some of their femininity and therefore will
become depressed. However, the womb is merely a muscle
and has no effect at all on feminine characteristics apart from
its relationship with menstruation. Unless the ovaries are
taken out at the same time there is no reason why you should

require HRT. If the ovaries are removed then HRT should not upset your diabetes unless of course you were taking more hormones than you were producing yourself until the operation. This could easily be put right by reducing the dosage or altering the preparation. The best person to discuss this with is your consultant. Make a list of the questions you want to discuss with him before you see him. Many patients find that what they wanted to discuss goes straight out of their mind as soon as they walk through his consulting room door. He will not be at all put off if you arrive with a list of questions. In fact, he will probably be impressed with your thoughtfulness.

25 *I have read in a magazine that the pill can now be taken by diabetics. My question is whether following this significant advance it can be hoped that hormone replacement therapy, which is widely available to non-diabetics during the menopause, may also become available to diabetics?*

Hormone replacement therapy for the menopause consists of small doses of oestrogens which are given to replace the oestrogens normally produced by the ovaries which at this time begin to decline, and if they decline rapidly can cause unpleasant symptoms. Replacement therapy is thus designed to allow a more gradual decline in circulating oestrogens. There is no reason why diabetics should not use this sort of hormone replacement therapy if the symptoms warrant it. Like the pill which also contains oestrogen, this sort of hormone therapy does often impose a slight increase in demand for insulin. A mild diabetic on diet alone or diet and tablets might possibly find that she cannot meet the increased demand for insulin without having supplementary insulin by injection but this would be very unlikely as the increased demand produced by oestrogens is so small. Similarly a diabetic already on insulin may occasionally experience an increased dose requirement. On balance, therefore, if the menopausal symptoms are sufficient to warrant hormone replacement therapy, which any way would be required only for a limited period, then the risk of causing a need for insulin injections in the diabetic who is not already on insulin would be small. This would not be of any importance if the diabetic was already on insulin.

Termination

26   Is diabetes grounds for termination of pregnancy?

Not unless your doctor considers that pregnancy would be detrimental to your health which may occasionally be the case. All the reasons for termination of pregnancy apply equally to diabetics as they do to non-diabetics.

27   Is it safe for a diabetic to have an abortion?

There is no added hazard to diabetics undergoing termination of pregnancy and care of the diabetes during this operation does not raise any special difficulties.

6

Pregnancy

Introduction

Pregnancy has been the first aspect of diabetic life where it has been shown without any doubt that poor blood glucose control is associated with many complications for both mother and child and that these complications are preventable by strict control. The outcome for diabetics who are pregnant and for the babies that they carry is directly related to how successful they are in controlling blood sugar concentration. If control is perfect from the moment of conception to delivery, then the risks of pregnancy to mother and baby are no greater than in non-diabetics.

We now know that poor control at the time the egg is fertilized (conception) can affect the way in which the egg divides and changes into the fetus (in which all organs and limbs are present but very small) in such a way as to cause congenital abnormalities (such as hare lip, contracture of the spine and holes in the heart). The risk of this happening can be reduced to a minimum and possibly even eliminated, by ensuring perfect diabetic control (normal HbA_1 levels) before getting pregnant.

For those who become pregnant when control is poor, there will be an increased risk of congenital abnormalities — some of which may be detectable by ultrasound early in pregnancy when termination is possible if a major defect is detected. When no defect is detected the outcome of the pregnancy will still be dictated by the degree of control during the 40 weeks of pregnancy and during labour and delivery. Modern antenatal care is usually shared between the diabetic specialist and the obstetrician, often at a joint antenatal clinic. Regular clinic attendance and strict compliance with diet, insulin and home blood glucose monitoring is sufficient to allow most diabetics to achieve perfect control (normal HbA_1 level) without the need for hospital admission. So long as control remains perfect and pregnancy progresses normally, there is no need for hospital admission. With the excellent control that is now possible, fetal development — monitored by regular ultrasound examinations — is usually normal and it is the authors' view that the pregnancy can be allowed to go to its natural 'term' (40 weeks). If spontaneous labour begins the procedure is no different from non-diabetics other than the continued need to keep the mother's blood sugar normal to prevent hypoglycaemia in the infant shortly after birth.

Diabetics are not immune to obstetric and antenatal complications and these will be treated in the same way as they would be in non-diabetics. When satisfactory diabetic control is not achieved at home, then admission to hospital becomes essential but there are very few mothers who cannot achieve and maintain normal blood sugar values as an out-patient, at least while they are pregnant. It is a remarkable example of the importance of motivation in the struggle for good diabetic control. The single-mindedness of the pregnant mother is able to cope with almost anything to protect the growing baby from harm. Sadly this motivation is often lost once the pregnancy is over and control slips back to where it was before.

There is no inherent reason why control is easier during pregnancy — the evidence strongly attributes this success to motivation — one has to realize that it should be possible to achieve this level of motivation in non-pregnant females (and even males!) since the rewards are just as immediate and tangible: good health and confidence in the future.

Genetics

1 If diabetes is known to be in the family can other members of the family take any preventative action?

The inheritance of diabetes is a complicated subject — indeed different sorts of diabetes appear to be inherited in different ways. For instance a tendency for one sort of diabetes (insulin dependent or juvenile onset) can be inherited, but only a small proportion of these people will go on to develop diabetes. One can now tell if these people at risk have inherited the relevant genes but even if they have, there is no way, as yet, of predicting their chances of developing diabetes. The commoner non-insulin dependent (or maturity onset) diabetes often treated by diet or diet and tablets is not associated with any known single gene abnormality but is thought to be strongly inherited — indeed when we have learnt more about it, it may well prove that there are several different sub-types at present not easily distinguished from one another — all inherited in different ways. We do know that many of these patients are overweight and that obesity not only makes diabetes worse but it may even lead to its appearance in susceptible people.

There is no really effective action other family members can take except to follow the usual health advice, keep physically active, eat a balanced diet and avoid obesity. It is worth bearing in mind the slight possibility that someone else in the family may become diabetic — especially if he or she ignores this advice — and test his or her urine as soon as he or she develops any symptoms which you may think relevant so that the diabetes can be detected and treated early on.

2 The man I am going to marry is a diabetic. Will there be any risk in having children?

If you are not a diabetic yourself and there is no diabetes in your family the risk of your children developing diabetes in childhood or adolescence, if the father is diabetic, are very small — probably no more than about 1 in 100. Provided you are both in good health it is certainly alright to have a family.

If you were diabetic and your fiancé were an insulin-requiring diabetic, then there would be increased risk of your children developing diabetes, although it is difficult to give a precise estimate; it is in the order of 1 in 10, or possibly even a 1 in 5 risk of them developing diabetes by the time they reach 70.

There is a rare form of non-insulin requiring diabetes in which there is a strong hereditary tendency. The risk of your children getting diabetes of this unusual kind would then be rather high but it is a mild form of diabetes and runs true to type throughout the generations.

The study of the inheritance of diabetes is a complicated subject and you would be well advised to discuss this further with your diabetic specialist or a professional genetic counsellor.

Management

3   *I am 25 years old and an insulin-dependent diabetic. My husband and I plan to start a family but first I would like to complete a 3-year degree course at university. By the time this course finishes I will be 29. Can you tell me if this will be too old to have a baby?*

You pose a difficult question as to the ideal age a diabetic should have a baby. The age of 29 is not too old to start a family but there are certain advantages in starting younger, particularly if you are a diabetic and if you plan more than one pregnancy. Starting a family may be hard work whether you are a diabetic or not. If you consider the additional difficulty of increasing age, I am sure you will understand why one normally recommends starting earlier rather than later.

It is of course difficult to give exact advice to individual people without knowing them personally and your clinic doctor who knows you well and your diabetes best is always the right person to talk to.

4   *I am worried that if I become pregnant whilst my
    husband's diabetes is uncontrolled the child will suffer —
    am I right?*

No. There is no known way in which poor control of your
husband's diabetes can affect the development of a child that
you will carry.

5   *When 7 months pregnant I developed diabetes. I had 8
    units of insulin a day. After my baby was born, I was
    tested and everything was normal so I discontinued
    insulin. I would now like another baby. My GP says I
    could become permanently diabetic. Another doctor,
    however, says this is very unlikely — please could you
    advise me?*

You suffered from gestational diabetes (that is, diabetes that
occurs during pregnancy and then goes away again when you
are not pregnant). The chances are that this will recur in
every subsequent pregnancy and you may well find that at
some stage it does not get better at the end of the pregnancy
and that you are then permanently diabetic. Even if you do
not have further pregnancies, you are a 'high risk' (greater
than 50:50) case for developing diabetes at some stage in the
future. Your pancreas produces enough insulin to cope with
every-day life but the extra demands of pregnancy are more
than it can manage, hence the need for extra insulin. You
should pay particular attention to your diet and fitness and
keep your weight at even slightly below your ideal weight
for height. The decision on whether to have further
pregnancies and inevitably putting yourself at risk of
developing permanent diabetes, is one that you alone can
take but you should be quite clear that you and your husband
understand the facts.

6   *When I had my first baby, I was in hospital for the last 2
    months of pregnancy and I was given a caesarian section
    after 36 weeks of pregnancy. My baby weighed 3.7 kg
    (8 lb 4 oz) even though it was 4 weeks early. During my
    most recent pregnancy I was allowed to go into labour
    which occurred at 39 weeks, the baby weighed 3.2 kg (7*

lb) and I spent absolutely no time at all in hospital other than to deliver the baby. My first child is 5 years old now and is very well and my new baby seems to be progressing very well. Why has there been such a big change in treatment?

The last 5 years has seen a dramatic change in our attitudes to the management of pregnancy in diabetics. We now know that it is good blood sugar control which is the most important goal to aim for during pregnancy and with home blood glucose monitoring this could be achieved in the majority of diabetics without the need for admission to hospital at any stage. It sounds as if during your first pregnancy your control was not as good as during the second one and that the early delivery by caesarian section was a result of the fact that the baby has already grown to 3.7 kg by 36 weeks and they are worried that it would become even bigger if left to 38 or 39 weeks. The heavier baby in the first pregnancy was because the high blood sugar you were running resulted in more fat being laid down on the baby to increase his weight. However, during your second pregnancy, when your diabetic control was clearly a good deal better, the baby grew at a more normal rate so that it was at the correct weight when you went into labour at the end of pregnancy.

7 *During my last labour I was given a drip and had an insulin pump up all day. Why was this necessary?*

Strict blood sugar control during labour is very important to ensure that you do not put your baby at risk from hypoglycaemia in the first few hours of life. If there is any possibility that your labour may end up with an anaesthetic (for example, for forceps delivery or possible caesarian section) then the simplest way to keep diabetes well controlled is with glucose being run into your circulation and matched with an appropriate dose of insulin. With the pump this means that should an emergency arise you will be immediately ready.

8 *During my pregnancy I found attending the antenatal clinic a nuisance and I did not like to keep my diabetes too well controlled because if I did I had many hypos. Labour and delivery seemed to go quite normally but my baby was rather heavy. He was 4.2 kg (9 lb 4 oz), and had to spend a long time in the Special Care Baby Unit because they said he was hypoglycaemic — how do I avoid all this trouble in my next pregnancy?*

If you want to go ahead and have further babies then it is essential that you change your attitude to attending the antenatal clinic and controlling your diabetes throughout the course of pregnancy. The trouble your baby had from hypoglycaemia was a reflection on the fact that the baby had been exposed to a very high glucose concentration in your body throughout pregnancy and has had to produce a lot of insulin from its own pancreas to cope with this extra load of sugar from you. Immediately after birth it no longer had the glucose coming from you but still had too much insulin of its own, hence the hypoglycaemia. You can prevent this risk in subsequent pregnancies by ensuring that your control is immaculate which will require you to attend the antenatal clinic on a regular basis and to do frequent blood glucose monitoring and to ensure that your control is excellent. If you can do this you should be able to eliminate any risk of hypoglycaemia in your baby.

9 *Breast feeding. Is it all right for me to breast feed my baby if my tests are positive?*

Breast feeding is generally encouraged these days and diabetics are also encouraged to do the same. There are no special difficulties in the diabetic and the presence of some sugar in the urine need not worry you too much provided that your diabetic control is not too bad. For the best results with breast feeding, a diet fairly high in calories is needed and you should keep a watchful eye on the diabetes, making appropriate adjustments to the insulin dose if necessary. If you find all this too much, it is obviously perfectly all right to bottle feed.

10 *I am married to a diabetic who takes insulin to control his diabetes. I have just become pregnant. What special things do I need to do during pregnancy to ensure that it goes smoothly and without complications?*

You need take no special precautions other than those taken by non-diabetics since the fact that your husband is a diabetic does not put your pregnancy at any particular risk. It is only when the mother is diabetic that the strict control and careful monitoring of control of blood glucose become essential.

11 *I have been told that I must keep my blood sugars as low as possible. Please tell me what 'low' is?*

Your blood sugars before meals should be between 3 and 6 mmol/l and 2 hours after meals no higher than 10 mmol/l.

12 *I am frightened of having hypoglycaemic attacks especially as I have been told to keep my blood sugars much lower. What should I do?*

There is no reason why you should have any hypoglycaemic attacks whilst pregnant, but all diabetics should be prepared for a 'hypo'. Carry glucose or dextrose or something like a mini Mars bar on you at *all* times. Most convenient are Dextrosol tablets — one of these raises the blood glucose by about 0.5 mmol/l, so you should take 2–4 for a 'hypo'.

13 *Do hypoglycaemic attacks during pregnancy harm the baby?*

No. There is no evidence to suggest that a very low blood sugar in the mother can harm the baby.

Complications

14 *My second son was born with multiple defects and has subsequently died. I have been an insulin-dependent diabetic for 14 years (since the age of 10). Are diabetics more likely to have an abnormal baby?*

The secret to a successful pregnancy in a diabetic is perfect blood sugar control starting before conception and lasting throughout pregnancy. There is good scientific evidence to suggest that multiple developmental defects are caused by poor control in the first few weeks of pregnancy and that the risk of this can be avoided by ensuring immaculate control at the time that the baby is conceived. The risks in terms of multiple congenital defects seem to be confined to the early stages of the pregnancy which is hardly surprising because this is the stage when the various components of the baby's body are beginning to develop and this is the stage where other illnesses such as German measles (rubella) also affect development.

Good control is also needed for the rest of the pregnancy because the gradual maturation and growth of the baby can be disturbed by poor control. In particular with poor control the baby grows rather faster than normal and is large in size although the development of the organs remains relatively immature in terms of their function. This does not happen with well-controlled diabetes. Because the baby is large the mother has to be delivered early and because the baby is immature it is susceptible to a number of added risks immediately after birth.

15   *My baby had difficulty in breathing in his first few days in the Special Care Unit. They said this was because of my poor diabetic control — why was this?*

It sounds as if your baby had what is called the respiratory distress syndrome (RDS) which occurs most commonly in premature babies. It occurs in babies of diabetic mothers where the baby has grown too quickly because of poor blood glucose control, and is born before it has become fully mature. It used to be a relatively common cause of death in babies of diabetic mothers but now because of stricter control and supervision the mother does not have to be delivered early. It is now uncommon and indeed can probably be completely prevented if patients control their blood glucose throughout pregnancy thus allowing the pregnancy to proceed for the normal 40 weeks.

16 *I had three hypoglycaemic comas when expecting my
son 11½ years ago and I wondered whether this could
have caused brain damage? As although he is bright and
is in the 'A' stream at school he does not seem to be able
to keep his work reasonable and presentable*

We are confident we can reassure you that your son has not
got brain damage. This rarely happens even to the diabetics
themselves and if you have managed to survive the comas
without brain damage then there was no risk to your child.

17 *I have read that the babies of diabetic mothers tend to
be fat and have lung trouble shortly after birth and also
be susceptible to hypoglycaemia (low blood sugar)
shortly after birth — is this true? And if so why does it
happen?*

We now know that if the mother runs a high blood sugar
throughout pregnancy, sugar gets across the placenta into
the baby's circulation and causes it to become fat. This is
because the baby's pancreas is still capable of producing
insulin even though the mother's cannot. As a result of this
the babies grow bigger during pregnancy than they should
do and delivery has to be carried out earlier than normal to
avoid obstruction of labour by the large baby. This used to
be carried out most commonly by caesarian section at about
36 weeks of pregnancy. One of the complications of this
method of delivery was the lung trouble in the babies, known
as the respiratory distress syndrome (RDS), caused by the
fact that the babies were born before the lungs were
properly developed. We now know that if the mother's blood
sugars are kept strictly within normal limits during
pregnancy, the babies do not grow faster than they should do
and that pregnancy can be allowed to continue for the
normal period of 40 weeks without the baby growing too big.
This avoids the risk of caesarian section in the majority of
patients and RDS is rarely seen because babies are fully
mature when they are born. The low blood sugar during the
first few hours after birth was a result of the fact that the
baby's pancreas had been producing a lot of insulin during
the pregnancy to cover the high blood sugar of the mother,

which was passed across the placenta to the baby. If the blood sugar is strictly controlled during the pregnancy and delivery, hypoglycaemia is seldom a problem.

18 *Are babies of diabetic mothers more likely to have jaundice?*

Babies born to diabetic mothers are likely to be jaundiced. This is partly because they tend to be born early. We do not know the reasons why the mature babies are jaundiced. The jaundice is usually mild and clears without treatment.

19 *I developed toxaemia during my last pregnancy and had to spend several weeks in hospital even though my diabetic control was immaculate. Luckily everything turned out alright and I now have a beautiful healthy son. Was the toxaemia related to me being a diabetic? And is it likely to recur in subsequent pregnancies?*

There seems to be some doubt as to whether diabetics are more prone to toxaemia or not. On balance most experts believe that they are not more likely to develop it. Regarding your second question, you are not more likely to get toxaemia in your future pregnancies, indeed the risk is less.

20 *During my last pregnancy I had hydramnios and my obstetrician said that this was because I was a diabetic. Is this true? And is there anything that I can do to avoid it happening in future pregnancies?*

Hydramnios is, I am afraid, more common with diabetic mothers and does appear to be related to how strictly you control the diabetes throughout pregnancy, so my advice to you is that, on future occasions, you can reduce the risk to an absolute minimum by ensuring that your HbA_1 and blood sugars are completely normal from the day of conception.

21 *During my recent delivery of my fourth child which went quite smoothly I had an insulin pump into a vein during labour. I had not had this in my previous three*

pregnancies, although I had been diabetic in all of them. Why did I need the pump this time?

We now know that it is important to keep the blood sugar in normal limits during labour to minimize the risk of the baby developing a low blood sugar (hypoglycaemia) in the first few hours after birth. This is most effectively and easily produced by the use of an intravenous insulin infusion combined with some glucose given as an intravenous drip. This means that the blood sugar can be kept strictly regulated at the normal level until delivery has been achieved and ensures that, should complications arise and something like a caesarian section be required, you are all ready immediately for an anaesthetic and operation.

22 *I have had a previous child that was delivered by caesarian section. Do I have to have a caesarian section with my next pregnancy?*

It all depends on why you had the caesarian section. If it was performed for an obstetric reason which is likely to be present in this pregnancy, then the answer is yes. If it was performed because the first baby was large or just because you are a diabetic, the answer could be no.

Some doctors do consider it safer to deliver women by caesarian section once the mother has had one. Others would allow you a 'trial of labour'. In other words, you would be allowed to start labour and, if satisfactory, you may be able to deliver your baby vaginally.

23 *My doctor tells me that I will have to have a caesarian section because my baby is in a bad position and a little large. What sort of anaesthetic is best?*

Nowadays approximately 50% of women have caesarian sections under epidural anaesthetic rather than under general anaesthetic. If you have an epidural anaesthetic your legs and tummy are made completely numb. This is done by injecting local anaesthetic solution through a needle into the spinal canal. You remain awake for the birth of your baby and therefore remember this event.

In most cases this kind of anaesthetic is better because your baby receives no anaesthetic and therefore is not sleepy.

If you are interested in having your baby this way, you must discuss it will your obstetrician.

Pre-antenatal

24 *I am a diabetic on tablets which I chose rather than insulin and I am pregnant again. As I have had a previous miscarriage I am worried about the chance of this recurring; both my husband and I smoke a lot. How can I make sure that this pregnancy is successful?*

Diabetic control certainly affects the outcome of pregnancy — better control leads to more successful pregnancies.

Good control should be established before conception if the pregnancy is planned, and is probably best maintained by either diet alone or if this fails, by diet with insulin. Currently we do not advise patients to take tablets throughout pregnancy although they do not harm the baby if they are inadvertently taken in the early part of pregnancy. The major hazards seem to be related to the immediate period after birth when the tablets which have previously crossed into the babies circulation stimulate insulin secretion causing hypoglycaemia in the baby.

It should also be said here that most diabetics of child-bearing age are already being treated with insulin, so that they are not normally faced with your decisions.

You obviously know already that smoking affects the baby — heavy smoking is associated with more miscarriages and smaller babies. In asking the question I suspect that you already know the correct answer: take insulin and do not smoke.

There is also more recently evidence to link even modest regular alcohol intake in pregnancy with unfavourable outcome as far as the baby is concerned. You should stop your drinking until the pregnancy is over.

25   *Why must I ensure that my diabetic control is perfect during pregnancy?*

To ensure that you reduce the risks to yourself and your baby to an absolute minimum. If you are able to achieve this degree of control from before the time of conception through to the time of delivery you can reduce the risks to your baby to those that are virtually indistinguishable from those of non-diabetics. On the other hand, if you do not control your diabetes properly and pay no attention to it the risk to the baby is very dramatically increased.

7

The young diabetic

Introduction

This chapter about diabetes in young people divides up
naturally into three main age groups: babies, children and
adolescents. The sections on babies and children consist of
questions asked by parents and the answers are naturally
directed at them. The section on adolescents is both for
young people and for their parents.

Apart from the experience of BDA camps, none of the
authors have actually lived with the daily problems of
bringing up a child with diabetes. However, we have listened
to hundreds of parents who have felt the despair of finding
that their child is diabetic, and then overcome their fears, to
allow their child to develop to the full. Mothers and fathers
usually end up by being especially proud of children who are
diabetic. We hope to pass on some of this experience to those
parents who are still at the frightened stage.

The diabetic baby

1 *My baby developed diabetes when she was 4 weeks old.
She is now 6 weeks and looks healthy but I would like
emergency advice in order to protect the baby's life.
What food and treatment should I give?*

You must be relieved that your baby is better now she has started treatment, but worried about the difficulties of bringing up a diabetic from infancy. Under the age of 1 year, diabetes is rare so you will not find many doctors with experience of this condition. However, the general principles are the same and there is no reason why she should not grow into a healthy young woman. The British Diabetic Association will let you have a booklet written by Dr Peter Swift for the parents of very young diabetic children. The BDA or your local clinic might also be able to get you in touch with other people who have had the same problem. Practical advice and reassurance from these would be more use than any theoretical advice.

Like all babies, your daughter will be fed on milk — breast or bottle. For the first 4 months frequent feeds are best — three hourly by day and four hourly by night. Bottle-fed babies usually need $2\frac{1}{2}$ oz of milk per lb body weight each day. Some babies grow rapidly and need more milk than this while others may need solids earlier than 4 months. This may be a help in diabetic babies as the solids will slow down the absorption of milk. It is important to wake young diabetic babies for a night feed to avoid night-time insulin reactions. If there is any doubt about this, a blood glucose check (while the baby is asleep) and an addition of 5–10 g carbohydrate will be reassuring.

2   *My little boy is nearly 1 year old and has been ill for a month, losing weight and always crying. Diabetes has just been diagnosed. Does this mean injections for life?*

Yes. I am afraid it does mean literally 'injections for life'. The thought of having to stick needles into a young child quite naturally horrifies parents. But, with loving care, explanations and playing games like injecting yourself and teddy bear (using a different needle) and perhaps some bribery, most children accept one or two injections as part of their normal day. Young children grow up knowing no other way of life and they often accept this treatment better than their parents. Encourage the child to help at injection time by getting the equipment ready or perhaps pushing in the plunger and pulling out the needle.

3   How can I collect urine for testing from my 18-month-old diabetic son? I have been given lots of different suggestions but none of them seem to work

It is not easy to get clean samples of urine from babies in nappies. Many infants will produce a specimen by reflex into a small potty when undressed. You can also squeeze a wet nappy directly into a urine testing stick. But be warned — washing powders or fabric softeners in the nappies alter the urine test result.

Diastix have the drawback that a large amount of ketones in the urine may interfere with the sticks so that a very sugary baby may only be thought to have a trace of sugar in the urine. Infants are much more likely than older people to have ketones in the urine. This is because they rapidly switch to burning up fat stores in the fasting state. It is important to check on ketones and try to keep the urine ketone-free, though you should not worry if ketones appear for a short time. Diabur-Test 5000 are a new urine stick which is not adversely affected by ketones. You should use Ketostix to test for ketones.

You will also have to do blood tests on your child. Parents expect these to be very painful to children but finger-prick blood tests are surprisingly well accepted by young people. They enable you to check accurately what is happening if your child feels unwell or looks ill. Urine tests only provide a guide about the diabetic state since the last urine specimen. The blood test confirms what is happening at that instant. It is the only reliable way of deciding whether your child is hypo or just tired and hungry. Blood sugars are also necessary to check the overall diabetic control and to help you decide on the dose of insulin if the blood sugar rises during an illness. Blood samples should be obtained with an Autolet (Owen Mumford Ltd, Brook Hill, Woodstock, Oxford) using the special platform for children.

4   My 2-year-old diabetic daughter makes an awful fuss about food. Meals are turning into a regular struggle. Have you any suggestions?

Food is of great emotional significance to all children. If meals are eaten without complaint, then both mother and child will have full stomachs and satisfied minds. All children go through phases of food refusal because of a need to show their growing independence, their ability to provoke worry or anger in parents and their attempts to manipulate the situation. Food leads to the well-known problem of the breakfast battleground which occurs in all families at some stage. The only way for the parent to win is to remain in control of the weapon. Usually when young children begin their negative phase (10–18 months), they dislike being told to leave the table and go away. They often return and accept food rather than remain alone and hungry.

The battle is even more difficult for the parents if the child is diabetic — the child has some explosive weapons! However, the parents must stay in control: try distracting attention away from food by toys, music, talk or their own relaxed approach to eating. You may have to send your child away from the table if he or she is refusing to eat properly. Hypoglycaemia often provokes hunger, and a couple of mild hypos due to food refusal is a small price to pay for better behaviour next time. Be prepared to modify the type of carbohydrate within reason if she consistently refuses the diet recommended by the hospital. Bread, potatoes, biscuits, fruit juices and even ice cream can be offered as alternatives.

5   *My 5-year-old son has been a diabetic since he was 18 months old and he is only 96 cm tall. I have been told that he is short for his age. The doctor says that poorly controlled diabetes could be slowing his growth. Is this true?*

The average height for a 5-year-old boy is 108 cm (3′ 6″), so your son is certainly short for his age. Having high sugar levels for several years could be the cause of this. If you now keep his diabetes under control and make sure that he has plenty to eat, he should grow rapidly and may even catch up with his normal height.

6 *My daughter is now 6 years old and has been diabetic for*
   4 years. She is on 12 units of Lente insulin, once a day.
   Her urine test in the morning is always 2% and the
   teatime test ¼%. My own doctor is satisfied with her
   test and says that negative tests in a child of this age
   means a risk of hypos. However, the school doctor says
   her diabetes is out of control and she should have two
   injections a day. What do you advise?

Until a few years ago most doctors did not try to achieve
close diabetic control in children. It was considered good
enough if the child felt well and was not having a lot of hypos.
The feeling nowadays is that good control *is* important to
allow normal growth and prevent long-term complications.
In the first place, you should start measuring your
daughter's blood glucose. This will tell you how serious is the
early morning high sugar and also whether she is running
the risk of a hypo at any other time of the day. It is likely
that she will need an evening injection to control the
morning blood sugar. It is true that keeping the blood sugar
down towards normal may make a hypo more likely. Mild
hypos do not cause any harm and even severe reactions do no
damage, except to the parent's confidence! You must not
worry about a few days or weeks of poor control; and you
will never achieve perfection in a little girl whose activity
and life-style is changing daily.

The diabetic child

7 *I have been told not to expect my daughter to be as tall*
   as she would have been if she had not been diabetic. Is
   this true? If so, what can I do to help her reach her
   maximum height?

Unless your daughter's diabetic control has been very poor,
there is no reason why she should not reach a normal height
without any special encouragement. We know of one 16-year-
old boy who is 6′ 2″ tall and has been diabetic for 10 years.
Diabetes does not necessarily stunt your growth.

8 *My 18-year-old son is only 5' 2" and very immature. I have heard that diabetics reach puberty a year or two later than anyone else. Will he grow later?*

If your son is sexually under-developed then he will certainly have a growth spurt when he goes into puberty. However, 5' 2" is very under-sized for a boy of 18. It *could* be poor diabetic control that has stunted his growth but there are other possible factors, including the physical stature of his father and yourself. If you are both of normal height, there could be some other medical reason for your son's short size. It would be worth consulting your GP or clinical doctor rather than blaming it automatically on diabetes.

9 *My son, aged 10, started insulin last year and his dose of insulin has gradually dropped until recently he has come off insulin completely and is on diet alone. Will he now be off insulin permanently?*

No. There is a 99.9% chance that he will have to go back on insulin. This so-called 'honeymoon period' (p.24) can be trying as it raises hopes that the diabetes has cleared up. Unfortunately, this never happens in young people.

10 *Are there any special schools for diabetic children?*

There are no special schools for diabetics and they would not be a good idea. It is most important that a young diabetic grows up in normal surroundings and is not encouraged to regard himself as 'different'. So he should go to a normal school and grow up in a normal family atmosphere.

11 *I think my newly diagnosed diabetic son is using his insulin injections as a way of avoiding school. I cannot send him to school unless he has his insulin but it sometimes takes ages before I can get him to have his injection. I have two younger children and a husband whom I also have to help to get to school and work. How should I cope with my temperamental son?*

You raise several related points. Firstly, you assume that he is using his insulin injections to avoid school. You may be right if he resisted going to school before becoming diabetic. In this case you should try the same tactics you used before. Alternatively, his dislike of school could be related to the diabetes; for example, an over-protective attitude by sports instructors, frequent hypos or embarrassment about eating snacks between meals. If you suspect such difficulties, a talk to your son and his form-master might clear the air.

He may be happy about school but actually fears his insulin injections so that things get off to a slow start in the morning. Problems with injections have been reduced with the introduction of plastic syringes with short, sharp needles, but some children focus their dislike for diabetes as a whole on the unnatural process of injecting themselves.

The BDA has produced a School Pack to help parents communicate with the school. It will contain a number of leaflets to be given to teachers and those responsible for diabetic schoolchildren. You should apply to the BDA for a copy of this publication.

12 When my son starts school, would it be better for him to return home for lunch or let him eat school dinners?

It depends largely on your son's temperament and attitude to school. Some 4 year olds skip happily off to their first day at school without a backward glance (much to their mother's chagrin), while other perfectly normal children make a fuss and have tummy aches at the start of school. Diabetes will tend to add to these problems. You will have to talk to the teachers and it would be worth asking their advice and making sure that someone will take the responsibility of choosing suitable food for your son — you cannot leave that to a 4- or 5-year-old child.

13 My 10-year-old son has recently been diagnosed diabetic. What is the best age for him to start doing his own injections?

The fear of injections loom large in a child's view of his own diabetes. Many children actually make less fuss if they do their own injections and most diabetic specialist nurses would encourage a 10 year old to do his own injections right from day one. I know a little girl who became diabetic at the age of 6 and who gave her own first injection without any fuss — and has been doing so ever since. Plastic syringes which can be reused take a lot of the horror out of injections.

If you do have an injection problem or if you want your son to have a good summer holiday, send him on a BDA holiday — you will find details in *Balance*.

14 *When I heard that I was to have a diabetic child in my class (I am a Junior School Teacher), I read all I could about diabetes. Most of my questions were answered but I cannot discover what to do if the child eats too much sugar. Will he go into a coma? If so, what do I do then?*

Eating sugar or sweets may make his blood sugar level rise in which case he may feel thirsty and generally off colour. Coma from a high blood sugar takes some time to develop and there is cause for concern only if he becomes very drowsy or starts vomiting. If this does happen, you should contact his parents. A child who is vomiting with poor diabetic control may need to go to hospital.

The most common sort of coma, which may occur over a matter of 10 minutes, is due to a hypo. In this case the blood sugar level is too low and he needs to be given sugar at once. The causes of hypo are delayed meals, missed snacks or extra exercise.

15 *Can I apply for an Attendance Allowance to look after my son who has frequent hypos and needs a lot of extra care?*

Some parents of children with extremely erratic diabetes have been granted an Attendance Allowance. However, the majority of diabetic children do not need 24-hour supervision and, therefore, an Attendance Allowance is not warranted. The BDA takes the official view that an allowance would only encourage your son to regard himself as disabled and the BDA does not support such applications.

*16 My little boy is diabetic and is always having coughs
and colds. These make him very ill and he always
becomes very sugary during each illness despite
antibiotics from my doctor. Could you please give me
some guidelines for coping with his diabetes during
these infections?*

Here are some guidelines:

1 *Insulin* — NEVER stop the insulin even if the child is
vomiting. During feverish illnesses the body often needs
more insulin, not less. During an illness it may be useful
to use only clear (short-acting) insulin. You may have to
give three or four injections a day as this is much more
flexible and you can respond more quickly to changes in
the situation. Give one-third of the total daily insulin dose
in the morning, as clear insulin only.

2 *Food* — Stop solid food but give sugar drinks for
example, Lucozade 60 ml (10 g) or orange squash with
three tablespoons of sugar (10 g). Milk drinks and
yoghurt are an acceptable alternative for ill children.
Aim to give 10–20 g every hour.

3 *Blood tests* — At midday, check the blood sugar and if it
is 13 mmol/l or more, give the same dose of clear insulin
plus an extra 2 units. Repeat this process every 4–6
hours, increasing the dose of insulin if the blood sugar
remains high. Once he is better, cut the insulin back to
the original dose.

4 *Ketones* — Check the urine for ketones twice daily. If
these are + + +, either your son needs more food or his
diabetes is going badly out of control.

5 *Vomiting* — Young diabetic children who vomit more
than two or three times should *always* be seen by a
doctor or specialist nurse to help supervise the illness.
They can become dehydrated in the space of a few hours
and if vomiting continues they will need fluid dripped
into a vein. Unfortunately, this means a hospital
admission.

*17 I am headmaster of a school for deaf children and one of
my pupils developed diabetes 2 years ago. Since then*

his learning ability has deteriorated, and I wondered if this had any connection with his diabetes?

No — diabetes in itself has no effect on learning ability and there are plenty of diabetic children who excel academically. Poorly controlled diabetes with a very high blood sugar could reduce his powers of concentration. Hypoglycaemic attacks are usually short lasting but he could be missing a few key items while his blood glucose is low and be unable to catch up. At a psychological level, the double handicap of deafness and diabetes could be affecting his morale and self-confidence. Perhaps he would be helped by meeting other diabetic boys of his age. This often helps children to realize that diabetes is compatible with normal life and activities.

18 *My son was recently awarded a scholarship to a well-known public school but when they found he was diabetic, he was refused admission on medical grounds. They can give no positive reason for this, and our consultant has tried hard to make them change their minds. Why should he be so penalized?*

This was a disgraceful decision based on old-fashioned prejudice. It looks as if nothing will make the school change its mind but I wonder if you told the British Diabetic Association about this matter. They might have brought more pressure to bear to make the school reconsider this extraordinary decision.

19 *How does my son tell his schoolfriends about his diabetes?*

It is important that your son tells his close friends that he is diabetic. He should explain about hypos and tell them that if he does behave in an odd way they should make him take sugar and he should show them where he keeps his supplies. If your son shows his friends how he measures his blood glucose they will almost certainly be interested in diabetes and be keen to help him with it. As he becomes older and spends more time away from home he will come to depend more on his friends.

20 *My 10-year-old son moves on to a large comprehensive school in a few months time. Up till now he has been in a small junior school where all the staff know about his diabetes. I worry that he will be swamped in the 'big' school where he will come across lots of different teachers who know nothing about his condition. Have you any advice on this problem?*

Moving up to a large comprehensive school is always a daunting experience and is bound to cause the parents of a diabetic child extra worry. The important thing is to go and talk to your son's form-teacher, preferably before the first day of term, when he will have hundreds of new problems to cope with. Assume that the teacher knows nothing about diabetes and try to get across the following points:

a My child needs daily insulin injections.
b He may need to eat at certain unusual times.
c Describe how your son behaves when hypo and emphasize the importance of giving him sugar. If he is hypo do not send him to the school office alone.
d Staggered lunch hours may be a problem as he may need to eat at a fixed time each day.
e Please let us know if he is going to be kept in late (e.g. for detention) as parents of diabetics tend to worry if their children fail to show up.
f Make sure all of his teachers know these facts.

The BDA supplies a school pack which should help explain diabetes to his teachers and it is especially important to speak personally to his sports and swimming instructors. If there are problems with the school over such things as sports, outings or school meals, your diabetic clinic may have a specialist nurse or health visitor who could go to the school and explain things. You will probably have to repeat this exercise at the beginning of every school year.

21 *What arrangements can I make with school about my 9-year-old daughter's special requirements for school dinners?*

It is first important to go and see the head teacher and preferably the caterer to explain that your daughter must have her dinner on time. Explain that she needs a certain amount of carbohydrate in a form that she will eat and that she must not be given puddings containing sugar. If the diabetic clinic has a specialist nurse or health visitor, she will be happy to go to the school and give advice.

Most parents of diabetic children solve the problem by providing a packed lunch. This means that you have more control over what your daughter eats and you can supply the sort of food she likes and that is good for her. When she goes on to secondary school she may be faced with a cafeteria system. This should allow her to choose suitable food but she may also choose unsuitable items (e.g. jam doughnuts).

22 *My son is diabetic. Can I allow him to go on school trips?*

In general the answer is yes, but for your own peace of mind you would want to be satisfied that one of the staff on the trip was prepared to take responsibility for your son. Day trips should be no problem as long as someone can be sure that he eats on time and has his second injection if necessary. At junior-school level, long trips away from home especially on the continent, could be more difficult and it really depends on your finding a member of staff that you can trust. They will need to keep an eye on your son and to know how to cope sensibly with problems like a bad hypo. Once in secondary school most diabetic children manage to go away on trips with the school, scouts or a youth group. Of course one of the adults in the party should be responsible, but as your son gets older he will be better able to look after himself. The British Diabetic Association has the following check-list for school trips and holidays:

a Identification necklace or bracelet.
b Glucose.
c Insulin, syringe, needles.
d Testing equipment for blood/urine.
e Food to cover journeys, with extra for unexpected delays.

This is part of a School Pack which is available from the BDA.

*23   My 10-year-old child has heard about BDA camps from
     the clinic. I am a bit worried about letting him go off on
     his own for 2 weeks. Do you not think that I should wait
     a few years before sending him to a camp?*

The BDA has been organizing holidays for children since the
1930s and it has become an enormous enterprise. Nearly
1000 children take part in these holidays each year, so in one
sense your son will not be on his own. Young children love
going on group holidays, and the fact of being with other
diabetics gives them a great sense of confidence — for once
the diabetics are not the odd ones out. The children learn a
great deal from each other and from the staff. Your son will
have an exciting holiday and you will have a few weeks off
from worrying about his diabetes.

24   Is it safe to let my little girl go to a BDA camp?

The Youth Department of the BDA has had years of
experience in running holidays for children. The average
camp consists of 30–35 children who are supervised by the
following staff:

> Warden, responsible for planning.
> Senior Medical Officer, who is experienced in diabetes.
> Junior Medical Officer.
> 2–4 nurses, usually with a special interest in diabetes
> and/or children.
> Three dietitians.
> 1–2 Deputy Wardens.
> Eight Junior Leaders, young adults with diabetes
> themselves, who give up 2 weeks to help.

The staff/child ratio is about 1:2 and there is always close
supervision on outings and all sports, especially swimming.

The diabetic adolescent

*25   My daughter and I are getting extremely anxious
     although our GP tells us there is nothing to worry
     about. She became diabetic when she was 14, 1 year*

after her periods had started. They stopped completely with the diabetes and have never started again, although we have now waited for 2 years. Is our GP right to be calm and patient, or are we right to be worried?

A major upset to the system such as diabetes may cause periods to stop in a young girl. It is a bit unusual for them not to reappear within 2 years and I would like to be certain that your daughter's diabetes is well controlled *and* that she is not underweight. Your doctor will be able to answer these two questions. If her diabetic control is good and she is of normal weight, then it would be reasonable to await another year or two before embarking on further investigations. There is a good chance that her periods will return spontaneously. If they do not return, nothing will be lost by waiting for another 2 years.

26 *I am nearly 16 and have not started menstruating yet. Is this because I am a diabetic? Since I was diagnosed, I have put on a lot of weight*

On average, girls with diabetes do tend to start their periods at an older age. I assume from your question that you are now overweight and this may be another cause for delay in menstruation. Presumably you have begun to notice other signs of puberty such as breast development and the growth of pubic hair. If so, you should make a determined effort to lose weight and control your diabetes carefully. This will include a reduction in your food intake and probably an adjustment in your dose of insulin. If, after another year, you have still not seen a period then you should discuss the matter with your doctor.

27 *My son has just heard that he will be going to university next year. While we are all delighted and proud of him, I worry because he will be living away from home for the first time. For the 7 years of his diabetes I have accepted most of the anxiety and practical arrangement of his meals and he has done his*

best to 'ignore' his diabetes. How is he now going to face it alone?

If your son is bright enough to get into university, he should be quite capable of looking after his diabetes. However, you are right to point out that your son's attitude towards his diabetes is also important. All mothers worry when their children leave home for the first time and it is natural for a diabetic child to cause extra worry. You can be sure, however, that the training you have given him over the years will prove beneficial. Most children like to spread their wings when first leaving home and you can expect a period of adjustment to his new responsibilities. Provided he realizes why you regard good diabetic control as important, he will probably become a model diabetic in good time. It would also be sensible for your son to contact the diabetic clinic in his university town, so that they can give support if necessary.

28 How does diabetes affect my prospects for marriage?

I have never heard a diabetic girl or boy complain that diabetes has put off potential marriage partners, though I suppose it could be used as an excuse if someone was looking for a convenient way out of a relationship.

If your diabetes has affected your own self-confidence and made you feel a second-class citizen, then you may sell yourself short and lose out in that way. You can be assured that diabetics make excellent husbands and wives.

29 I am an insulin-dependent diabetic and have recently made friends with a super boy but am frightened that he will be put off if I tell him I am a diabetic. What should I do?

It would have been better to tell your new boyfriend at the beginning. However, you have obviously found this a problem or you would not be asking the question. There is no need to broadcast the fact that you have diabetes. It would be possible to conceal diabetes completely from a close companion, though sooner or later he will inevitably discover the truth.

Once you get to know him better your best plan would be to drop a few hints about diabetes without making a song and dance about it. If the relationship grows, you will want to share each other's problems — including diabetes. I have never known a serious relationship break up because of diabetes.

30 My 15-year-old son developed diabetes at the age of 12. Initially he was sensible about his diabetes but recently he has become resentful, saying that he is different from everyone else and blaming us for his disease. What do you suggest?

You must first realize that most diabetics of all ages (and their parents) feel resentful about this disease which causes so much inconvenience in a person's life. Many 12-year-old children conform with their parent's wishes and generally do as they are told. However, by the age of 15 other important pressures are beginning to bear on a developing young person. In the case of a boy, the most important factors in life are probably (1) his friends and (2) girls. While you as parents are prepared to make allowances and provide special meals, etc., most young men want to be gregarious and do not wish to appear 'different'.

At the Firbush camp (see p.268) comprising of hand-picked, well-adjusted young adults with diabetes, the organizers were horrified to discover how angry the young people felt about their condition. Of course this anger will often be directed at the parents. We can only give advice in general terms which apply to most adolescent problems:

a   Keep open lines of communication.
b   Boost his self-esteem by giving praise where praise is due — even if your own self-esteem is taking a hammering.
c   Allow your son to make his own decisions about diabetes. If you force him to comply, he will simply avoid confrontation by deceiving you.
d   Remember that difficult adolescents usually turn into successful adults.

*31 Our 14-year-old daughter has had diabetes for 4 years
and until recently has always been well controlled. Now
it is difficult to get her to take an interest in her
diabetes and she has stopped taking blood tests. At the
last clinic visit, the doctor said that her HbA₁ was very
high and he thought she was probably missing some of
her injections. I really do not know what to do*

There is no simple answer to these questions concerning
human behaviour. First I would wonder about your
daughter's behaviour in the clinic. She might be prepared to
talk to the doctor more openly if you were not there.
However, I am not trying to suggest that a complex situation
like this can be solved by a few minutes in the doctor's office.
Your daughter is beginning to learn how to cope
independently with her own condition, and this is bound to
involve some experiments to find out how far she can go. To
repeat some advice from a previous question: remember that
nearly all adolescents turn into well-adjusted adults. Keep
talking to her about her diabetes but avoid nagging. Ask
your daughter how she feels about injections and *listen* to
the answer.

8

Long-term complications

Introduction

Before insulin was discovered diabetics did not survive long
enough to develop diabetic complications as we know them
today. In the early days after the great discovery, it was
commonly believed that insulin cured diabetes. We are now
in a better position to realize that although insulin produced
nothing short of miraculous recovery in those on the verge of
death from diabetic coma, and allowed them to return to a
full, active and enjoyable life, it is no cure for the condition.
But used properly insulin results in full health and activity
and a long life.

The life expectancy of diabetics has increased
progressively since insulin was first used in 1922 and there
are now many hundreds (and probably thousands) of patients
who have successfully completed 50 years of insulin
treatment. Increased longevity has brought with it a number
of the so-called 'long-term complications', some of which
(such as heart disease and gangrene of the legs) occur
commonly in non-diabetics and are generally considered to
be inevitable consequences of ageing (we all have to die
sometime!). Others are not seen in non-diabetics. These
conditions are therefore considered the 'long-term complications' specific to diabetes; the three most important are

retinopathy (eyes), neuropathy (nerves) and nephropathy (kidneys).

Diabetic retinopathy can lead to loss of vision and indeed is now the commonest cause of blindness registration in people under 65 in the United Kingdom. Fortunately, it only leads to visual loss in a small proportion of diabetics. Diabetic nephropathy can cause kidney failure and is now the commonest reason for referral for renal dialysis and transplantation in the UK and Europe in young people, although again it only occurs in a very small number of diabetic patients. Diabetic neuropathy, by leading to loss of feeling, particularly in the feet, makes affected patients very susceptible to infections and occasionally gangrene with the subsequent need for an amputation. It can also cause impotence.

It is not surprising that diabetic patients dread the thought of diabetic complications. In the past they worried about them but never mentioned them or asked questions about them since they were subject to some kind of 'taboo', which meant that they were only for discussion between doctors and not between doctor and patient.

Today patients rightly demand to know more about their condition ('whose life is it anyway?') and the majority now find out about the dreaded 'complications' very soon after they are diagnosed as diabetic. There are so many 'old wives' tales' circulating about diabetic complications. It is perhaps *the* most important area in diabetic counselling where the *facts* rather than opinions must be stated.

Although medical science has made impressive progress since the discovery of insulin there is still a long way to go and the absolute proof that good blood sugar control in diabetic patients will prevent the complications developing has not yet been made. The scientific evidence from studies of experimental diabetes in animals is very strongly in favour of this, however, and all the evidence from humans is in keeping with this. We believe that the specific diabetic complications are a direct result of a raised blood sugar level over many years and that they are all preventable by maintenance of normal blood glucose (and HbA_1) values.

General questions

*1   Can a diabetic who is controlled only by diet suffer from
    diabetic complications?*

Complications may occur in any type of diabetic. The cause
of diabetic complications is not well understood, although
bad control of diabetes is the most important predisposing
factor. The duration of diabetes is also important —
complications are rare in the first few years of the disorder
and occur more commonly after many years.

Diabetics treated with diet alone are usually diagnosed in
middle or late life. At the time their diagnosis is made, the
disease may have been present for a long time, often many
years, without the person having any knowledge of it, and
therefore without any attempt being made to control it.
Thus it is not surprising that complications can occur in some
diabetics even when they are treated with diet alone. Good
control in these patients is clearly just as important as in
insulin-dependent diabetics.

*2   Can bad sight be due to diabetes and if so how does it
    develop? And is there any connection between diabetes
    and kidney failure?*

You ask two important questions here and the answer to
both is yes — that is, diabetes can cause deterioration of
eyesight and it can lead to kidney failures.

With regard to eyesight it is necessary to remember that
acute changes of diabetic control both when deteriorating or
when improving can cause temporary blurring of vision.
Cataract is a little commoner in diabetics compared with non-
diabetics, but fortunately this cause of failing vision can
usually be treated by operation. Damage to the retina (back
of the eye) caused by diabetes is called retinopathy. It occurs
to a mild degree, after many years of diabetes, in many but
not all diabetics, and to a severe degree threatening vision in
only a few. It can take different forms and there are various
reasons why blindness sometimes occurs, the commonest of
these being haemorrhage (bleeding). Preventative treatment
for some kinds of retinopathy is now possible, and your eyes

are examined from time to time at the Diabetic Clinic to discover whether you require this.

Kidney failure is due to damage of the kidneys by the diabetes but is fortunately very rare.

With regard to both eye and kidney problems it is important to remember two things:

a Diabetic eye and kidney disease are commoner after years of bad diabetic control. Control is most important for prevention of complications and all diabetics should pay great attention to this.

b There are many kinds of both eye and kidney disease which affect diabetics and non-diabetics alike. The proper diagnosis and treatment always needs to be made by a specialist.

3 *My child has been diabetic for 3 years and I am trying to find out more about the disease. I recently read a book which said that some diabetics may suffer from coronary thrombosis or go blind. I do not know if this is true and find it very upsetting. Surely they should not be allowed to write such things in books that diabetics might read?*

You raise an interesting matter. Diabetes was almost always fatal within 1 or 2 years of diagnosis until the outlook was revolutionized by the discovery of insulin. None the less, it still required a lot of work and experimental development in the manufacture of insulin before a diabetic was able to lead an almost normal life, with the aid of one or two insulin injections a day.

After several years it became obvious to doctors that some diabetics were developing what we now call 'chronic complications'. It was clear that these took many years to develop. This became the object of a massive research drive, requiring the investment of much effort and entailing many years of work by doctors and other scientists. We now understand how some of these complications occur, and we know how to treat them if they occur. We realize that strict diabetic control is essential in their prevention. For this reason, all doctors and other medical personnel treating diabetics spend much of their time and effort trying to help patients improve their control and keep their blood sugars as near normal as possible. These complications do not occur in all diabetics by any means, though nowadays, when diabetics are living longer than ever before, the complications are becoming more important.

You ask whether facts like these should be made available to diabetics; the majority of patients like to be correctly informed about their condition, its management and its complications. Modern treatment includes increasing frankness between doctors and patients in discussing all aspects of the condition. A recent survey among our own diabetic patients showed that the majority demanded to be told the facts about complications.

4 *What are the complications and what should I keep a look-out for to ensure that they are picked up as soon as possible?*

The complications 'specific' to diabetes are known as retinopathy, neuropathy and nephropathy. Retinopathy means diabetic damage to the retina at the back of the eye. Neuropathy means damage to the nerves which can affect nerves supplying any part of the body. However, this is generally referred to as either 'peripheral' when affecting nerves supplying muscles and skin, or 'autonomic' when affecting nerves supplying organs such as the bladder, the bowel and the heart. Nephropathy is diabetic damage affecting the kidney which in the first instance makes it more leaky so that albumin appears in the urine; at a later stage it may affect the function of the kidney and in severe cases lead to kidney failure.

The best way of detecting them early is to attend your doctor or clinic for regular review. This is one of the reasons for regular attendance at the Diabetic Clinic so they can be picked up at an early stage and where appropriate, treatment instigated.

Prevention is, however, clearly better than treatment and we believe that if you can control your diabetes properly you will not be liable for these complications.

5 Is it possible to avoid complications in later life? If so, how?

Yes. We believe that all diabetics could avoid complications if they were able to control their diabetes perfectly from the day they were diagnosed as diabetics, and there are now many people on record who have gone 50 years or more with insulin-treated diabetes who are completely free from any sign of complication. The best advice to give you on how to avoid them is to take the control of your blood sugar and diabetes seriously from the outset and to attend regularly for review and supervision with somebody experienced in the management of patients with diabetes. Focus on learning how to look after yourself in such a way that you can achieve and attain a normal HbA_1 level (p. 129). If you can do that and keep the HbA_1 result normal you can look forward to a life free from the risk of diabetic complications.

6 To what extent are the complications of diabetes genetically determined?

This is a difficult question to answer. Most specialists believe that there is a hereditary factor which predisposes some patients to develop complications and makes others relatively immune from complications but so far scientific evidence to prove this is not very strong.

7 What is the expected life span of someone with insulin-dependent diabetes and why?

The life span depends to a great extent on how old the patient is when the diagnosis is made. The older the patient at the time of diagnosis the closer the life span is to that of non-diabetics. Looking back to the past we know that when diabetes was diagnosed in early childhood then the life span in insulin-dependent diabetics was generally reduced, mainly because of premature deaths from coronary attacks and kidney failure. We know, however, that the life span of diabetics has got progressively better with improvements in medical care and we have every reason to believe that the life expectancy of a child diagnosed as a diabetic in 1984 is longer than ever previously possible and may be nearly as good as that of a non-diabetic child from the same background. We know that longevity is greatest in diabetics who make regular visits to their clinic and who keep themselves under strict control and that those who die prematurely are more likely to be those who do not attend clinic regularly, are not being supervised adequately and do not control themselves well.

8 *My diabetic specialist has said that it does not follow that unstable diabetics get all the side-effects and ill health in their later life, often evidently well-controlled diabetics became ill and unbalanced diabetics remained reasonably healthy. Is this really true?*

There is an element of truth in the statement that you report but the word 'often' should be replaced by 'very occasionally' and the statement should read 'well-controlled diabetics rarely become ill and develop side-effects whereas unstable and unbalanced diabetics often develop ill health and side-effects in later life'.

9 *I am controlled by diet only but have a few side-effects and wonder whether they are complications? They are buzzing in the ears (tinnitus) and inflammation of the vulva and cystitis*

Buzzing in the ears (tinnitus) has probably nothing to do with diabetes. The inflammation of the vulva and cystitis suggests that you still have a lot of sugar in your urine and that your diabetes needs to be brought under control. These are not long-term complications but short-term complications of poor diabetic control.

10 *I have been a diabetic for several years and have recently developed severe chaps on the lips and on my fingers — what is this due to?*

This has nothing to do with diabetes and there are many possible causes. You should see your GP for advice and treatment.

11 *For the last 2 years my cheeks have become increasingly hollow although my weight is static — is this due to my diabetes?*

Quite a lot of middle-aged and elderly people become thin faced and gain wider hips irrespective of whether they have diabetes or not.

However, there is a rare form of diabetes called lipoatrophic diabetes, and this could possibly be the explanation for the hollowing of your cheek. This is not a recognized complication of diabetes but a rather rare and unusual form of the condition.

Eyes — see also p.136

12 *I had a tendency towards short-sightedness before being diagnosed as a diabetic. Is this likely to increase my chances of developing eye complications later on?*

Short-sightedness makes not the slightest difference to developing diabetic eye complications, although it has been said that those with severe short-sightedness may actually be less, rather than more, prone to retinopathy. Vision may vary with changes in diabetic control. Severe changes in blood sugar can alter the shape of the lens in the eye and thus alter its focussing capacity. It is therefore common in those with a high blood sugar (i.e. with poor control) to have difficulty with distant vision — a situation which changes completely when diabetes is controlled and blood sugar reduced. When this occurs, vision changes again, so that a person experiences difficulty with near vision and therefore with reading. This can be rather frightening at least until it is understood. After 2 or 3 weeks, vision always returns to the state it was in before diabetes developed.

13 *A friend has told me that on a recent TV programme it was stated that diabetics over 40 years of age were likely to become blind. This has horrified me because my 9-year-old son is diabetic and unfortunately some of*

*his schoolfriends have now told him about the pro-
gramme. What can I say to reassure him?*

Some damage to the eyes (retinopathy) occurs quite
commonly after more than 20 years of diabetes. Retinopathy
is, however, usually slight and does not affect vision. Only a
very small proportion of diabetics actually go blind, probably
no more than 7% of those who have had diabetes for 30
years. Because of the tremendous advances that have
occurred in diabetes over the last 30 years, this proportion of
diabetics with visual problems will be much smaller when your
son has had diabetes for 30 years. The figure is likely to be
smaller in well-controlled diabetics and larger in those who are
always badly controlled.

We have every reason now to believe that control of
diabetes influences the development of diabetic complications including retinopathy. That is why doctors and
their diabetic patients are together striving harder than
ever to maintain good control by urine tests and blood sugar
measurements. The aim of good control is of course to
eliminate all symptoms and to keep diabetics feeling well as
well as to avoid the long-term complications. To achieve good
control diabetics need to keep to a steady diet and take
regular insulin injections. Most diabetics are treated with
two injections a day although a few may take three or more,
in order to achieve good control. There is also a suggestion
that smoking may influence the development of retinopathy
so do your best to ensure that your son does not take up
smoking. I hardly need to mention all the other reasons why
smoking is best avoided.

*14   Can I wear contact lenses and if so would you
recommend hard or soft ones?*

The fact that you are a diabetic should not interfere with
your use of contact lenses or influence the sort of lens you
are given. Of greater importance in the choice of type would
be local factors affecting your eyes and vision and the correct
person to advise you would be an ophthalmologist or
qualified optician specialized in prescribing and fitting
contact lenses. It might be sensible to let him know that you
are diabetic and you must follow the advice you are given,

particularly to prevent infection; but this applies to diabetics and non-diabetics alike.

15 Are flashes of light and specks across one's vision symptoms of serious eye trouble with diabetic people?

Although diabetics do get eye trouble, flashing lights and specks are not usually symptoms of this particular problem. You should discuss it with your own doctor, who will want to examine your eyes in case there is any problem.

16 Why does diabetes affect the eyes?

A simple question but a difficult one to answer. Current research indicates strongly that it is excess glucose in the bloodstream that directly damages the eyes mainly through affecting the lining of the small blood vessels that carry blood to the retina. The damage to these vessels seems to be directly proportional to how high the blood sugar is and how long it has been increased. This is the reason why we all believe that this can be avoided by bringing the blood sugar down to normal.

17 What causes cataracts in diabetes?

Cataracts occur in non-diabetics as well as diabetics and as such are not necessarily a specific complication of diabetes. There is a rare form of cataract that can occur with very badly controlled diabetes in childhood; this is known as a 'snowstorm' cataract from its characteristic appearance to the specialist. The normal common variety of cataract which occurs in diabetics is exactly the same as that occurring in non-diabetics although it may occur at a slightly earlier age in patients with diabetes. It is really due to the ageing process affecting the substance that the lens of the eye is made of. It begins to develop wrinkles and becomes less clear than it was until eventually it becomes so opaque that it is not possible to see properly through it.

18 Is a diabetic cataract different from an ordinary cataract?

There is a cataract which occurs only in diabetics, the so-called 'snowstorm' cataract (see previous question) but this is rare. The common cataract that diabetics suffer from is exactly the same as those suffered in non-diabetics.

19   Please could you tell me what microaneurysms of the eye are?

Microaneurysms are little balloon-like dilations in the very small capillaries of the blood vessels supplying the retina at the back of the eye. They are one of the earliest signs that the high blood sugar has damaged the lining to these capillaries. As such they do not interfere with vision but give an early warning that retinopathy has begun to develop. There is some evidence to suggest that these can get better with the introduction of perfect control whereas at later stages of diabetic retinopathy reversal is not usually possible. Anyone who has microaneurysms must have regular eye checks so that any serious developments are detected at an early stage.

20   Can photocoagulation or laser treatment damage the eyes?

The strict answer to this is yes but uncommonly. Occasionally the lesion produced by the photocoagulation treatment can spread and affect vital parts of the retina which can interfere with vision. Normally treatment is confined to the bits of the retina which do not have a noticeable effect on vision other than perhaps to narrow the field of view slightly. Photocoagulation can also occasionally result in rupturing of a blood vessel and haemorrhage and after lots of photocoagulation there is a slight risk of damage to the lens causing a type of cataract.

21   Is glaucoma related to diabetes?

Yes. Although glaucoma can occur quite commonly in non-diabetics there is a slightly increased risk in diabetics. This is usually confined to those who have advanced diabetic eye problems (proliferative retinopathy).

Occasionally the eye drops that are put in your eyes to dilate the pupil to allow a proper view of the retina can precipitate an attack of glaucoma. The signs of this would be pain in the affected eye together with blurring of vision coming on some hours after the drops have been put in. Should this occur you should seek *urgent* medical advice either from your own doctor or from an accident and emergency department or your local hospital because this is reversible with rapid treatment but can cause serious damage if not treated.

22 *What is the difference between light coagulation and laser beam treatment for diabetic eye disease?*

Light coagulation (xenon arc coagulation) was the first form of light treatment produced for the treatment of diabetic retinopathy. It has been largely superseded by laser beam treatment. The principle of both forms of treatment is exactly the same but the size of the lesion produced is very much smaller with the laser than it is with the xenon arc. This is generally an advantage unless there are extensive areas of the retina which require treatment when the xenon arc is sometimes preferable. The laser can often be given with simple local anaesthesia to the eye whereas the xenon arc may require either a more complicated local anaesthetic or a general anaesthetic.

23 *Every time I receive my copy of* Balance, *the diabetic newspaper, I have the impression that the print gets smaller. Is this true or is there something wrong with my eyes? If my eyesight is getting worse then how can I go on reading* Balance?

I am afraid that eyesight does tend to deteriorate with age whether one is diabetic or not. The first thing to do is to visit your optician and get your eyesight checked to see if it can be improved with glasses. This may be all that is required. For people who are unfortunate and suffer from retinopathy to the degree that reading becomes impossible there are things that can help. *Balance*, for example, is available to members of the British Diabetic Association as a cassette recording and this service is free of charge. To satisfy post office regulations, though, you have to have a certificate of blindness before the cassette can be sent to you. Books in large type can be obtained from most public libraries or from:

Ulverscroft Books
The Green, Bradgate Road, Anstey, Leicester LE7 7FW
Telephone: 053 721 4325.

They print all types of books, including fiction and non-fiction. The Royal National Institute for the Blind also has a talking book service which is excellent.

Feet (chiropody and footwear) — see also p.139

24   What are the signs that diabetes is affecting our feet?

There are two major dangers from diabetes which may affect the feet. The first is due to diminished blood supply from arterial thickening. This leads to poor circulation with cold feet even in warm weather and cramps in the calf on walking (intermittent claudication). This is not a specific complication of diabetes and does occur quite commonly in non-diabetics. The major problem here is arterial sclerosis and smoking is a more important cause of this than diabetes. In severe cases this can progress to gangrene. The other way that diabetes can affect the feet is through damage to the nerves (neuropathy) which results in diminished sensation. This can be quite difficult to detect unless the feet are examined by an expert. The danger is that any minor damage to the foot, be it from a cut or abrasion or tightly fitting shoe, will not cause the usual painful reaction so that damage can result from continued injury or infection spreading. It is important that you should know whether the sensation in your feet is normal or impaired. Make sure you ask your doctor this at your next clinic review.

25   My daughter is diabetic and often walks barefoot around the house. Shall I discourage her from doing this?

It is well known that diabetics are prone to problems with their feet, which are, for the most part, due to carelessness and can be avoided. The reasons these problems occur is probably because, with increasing duration of diabetes, sensation in the feet tends to be a bit dulled. Most diabetics are unaware of this at the time and this is the source of danger — since to the unwary, damage to the feet is the first indication of the problem. By then it may be too late!

Damage to the feet easily occurs because poor foot sensation diminishes awareness of even minor injuries. The sources of trouble are many — unsuitable shoes featuring high among them. Other causes include rubbing from tight shoes (especially new ones); nails or stones in the shoes; walking barefoot and stepping on nails or other sharp objects; burns on the toes from hot water bottles or falling asleep too close to a fire; careless chiropody or, worst still, self-inflicted wounds from badly performed 'operations' on the feet with dirty instruments. Most foot problems are due to these causes and therefore it is obvious that most of them could be avoided.

For proper care of your feet *do* wash and dry your feet well every day, change your socks or stockings daily, see that your shoes are not too tight and check the insides for nails or stones and see a chiropodist regularly. *Do not* walk barefoot, sit too close to a fire or radiator, use a hot water bottle in bed, neglect even slight injuries or attempt your own chiropody (instead you should see a chiropodist).

The dangers to the feet of diabetic children are really very slight — but it is obviously right to train your daughter with the right habits at an early stage. I suggest that you should discourage her from walking about barefoot — but do not make a major issue out of it.

26 *Now that it is winter what special care should I take of my feet?*

One should not allow common sense to be undermined by unnecessary anxieties, but diabetics must take special care of their feet.

In a few instances diabetics who have had the condition for a long time may develop neuropathy and may lose some sensation in their feet. If this happens they do not feel the discomfort others might experience if their shoes were too tight or if a hard piece of leather rubbed the feet causing a blister or if a badly cut toenail rubbed and damaged an adjacent toe. The foot may become infected and difficult to treat.

In older diabetics the blood supply to the feet may not be as abundant as in non-diabetics and this will make the feet more vulnerable to damage by severe cold, trauma or infection.

What would be a minor cut in a non-diabetic's foot could be serious in a diabetic, particularly if the injury is not treated promptly.

Winter is cold and wet so we tend to wear warmer thick clothing. A pair of shoes which may be comfortable in the summer may be unpleasantly tight when worn with thick woolly stockings. This may damage the feet and also make them more sensitive to the cold. It could numb sensation completely. All these effects will be accentuated if your feet become wet. Make sure your shoes or boots are comfortable, fit well, and allow room for you to wear an adequately thick pair of socks, preferably made of wool or other absorbent material. Use weatherproof shoes, overshoes or boots if you are going to be out for any length of time in the rain or snow — and dry your feet carefully if they get wet. Do not put your cold — and slightly numb — feet straight onto a hot water bottle or near a hot fire because you may find that when the feeling comes back the heat was excessive.

There is little use in wearing warm socks and comfortable weatherproof shoes if you are otherwise exposed to the cold, so always wear warm clothes (see foot care rules p.142).

27   How can one give continual protection to one's feet?

It is extremely difficult. If the sensation is normal then by and large you have very little need to worry but if there is even slight numbness of the feet you should be continually vigilant and seek the advice of another to inspect the bits that you find difficulty in seeing. If the circulation is poor go to great lengths to keep your feet warm and well protected.

28   *I have suffered from foot ulcers for many years and would be grateful if you could suggest a cleaning fluid*

You should not attempt treatment of these yourself and should seek medical advice and expert chiropody. Foot ulcers in diabetics are most often associated with loss of sensation in the feet (neuropathy) and you need to have your feet examined by your specialist and find out whether you have loss of sensation. If this is the case then you need to attend for regular chiropody and to learn all the ways of avoiding trouble once sensation has become impaired (p.142).

29   *Please could you comment on the suitability of Scholl ingrowing toenail treatment for diabetics*

It all depends on whether the sensation and blood supply to your feet is normal. If it is normal then you can probably use the preparations as safely as non-diabetics. If, however, there is any question of the blood supply or nerve supply to your feet being compromised you should avoid it and seek expert advice from the clinic or your chiropodist.

30   *I have recurrent troubles with athlete's foot, which seems to recur whatever I do — is this because I am a diabetic? Do I have to be particularly careful with creams to treat this?*

Athlete's foot is due to a fungus infection. It is common in young people but diabetics do not seem to be unduly prone to it. The reason it keeps recurring is probably because you have not completely eradicated it. You should make sure that your doctor knows about this and gives you a prescription for an antibiotic which will eliminate the infection.

There are no particular risks for diabetics from the creams for athletes foot.

Kidneys

31 Why does diabetes sometimes affect the kidney and if it does how is it revealed?

There are several ways in which diabetes may affect the kidney. Firstly if there was a lot of sugar in the urine this predisposes you to infection which can spread from the bladder up to the kidneys (cystitis and pyelonephritis). Occasionally chronic kidney infections can produce very little in the way of symptoms and only be revealed by routine tests. In long-standing and poorly controlled diabetics high blood glucose can affect the small blood vessels supplying the kidney in the same way as it may affect the small blood vessels supplying the retina of the eye. This does not produce any symptoms but will be picked up on a routine urine test carried out at the Diabetic Clinic. Occasionally, massive amounts of albumin are lost in the urine which may make the urine froth and lead to accumulation of fluid in the body and the development of swelling around the ankles (oedema). For patients who have had long-standing kidney problems kidney failure may eventually develop. This is usually picked up on blood tests and urine tests many years before the symptoms develop.

32 Are diabetics with kidney failure suitable for dialysis and transplantation?

Yes. The majority of diabetics who are unfortunate enough to end up with kidney failure are suitable for both forms of treatment.

Dialysis (or chronic renal replacement therapy) is of two major types. The older type is chronic haemodialysis where the blood is washed in a special machine twice a week. The more recent type of dialysis is known as CAPD (Chronic Ambulatory Peritoneal Dialysis) where fluid is washed in and out of the abdomen on a daily basis. Diabetics seem to be rather good at this, it seems to be suitable for the patients with diabetes and is in many ways simpler and cheaper than haemodialysis. Eventual transplantation is the aim of most dialysis programmes but the supply of suitable kidneys is a limiting factor here. The source of kidneys is either from people dying accidentally who have donated their kidneys ('cadaver kidneys') or from live related donors who have agreed to give one of their two normal kidneys, usually to a relative suffering from kidney failure. A normal person can manage perfectly well with one kidney without any shortening of life provided that kidney does not get damaged. The donor of course will have to have an operation and will be slightly more vulnerable as a result because he will have only one kidney to rely on instead of two.

33 *I was found to have protein (albumin) in my urine when I last attended the Diabetic Clinic — what does this mean?*

If it was only a trace of protein if may mean nothing but you should get your urine checked again to make sure it remains clear. If it is a consistent finding it may indicate that you have an infection in the bladder or kidney (cystitis or pyelonephritis) or it could indicate that you have developed a degree of diabetic nephropathy (kidney damage). There are innumerable other causes of protein (albumin) in the urine and this is not necessarily related to the fact that you are a diabetic. If it is a consistent finding it will usually need to be investigated and you should ask your doctor to keep you informed of the results of the investigation.

Nerves

34 *I have been a diabetic on insulin for 3 years. Eighteen months ago I started to get pains in both legs and could barely walk. Despite treatment I am still suffering. Can you tell me what can be done to ease this pain?*

There are many causes of leg pains, and only one is due specifically to diabetes. This is a particularly vicious form of neuritis — in other words, a form of nerve damage which causes singularly unpleasant pain, chiefly in the feet or thighs, or sometimes both. The pain sensation is either one of pins and needles, or constant burning, and is often worse at night causing lack of sleep. Contact from clothes or bedclothes is often acutely uncomfortable. Fortunately this form of neuritis is rather uncommon and always disappears, although it may take many months before doing so. Good control of the diabetes is important and helps to alleviate the symptoms and speed recovery. Relief is otherwise obtained by good pain killers, as recommended by a doctor, and sometimes assisted by sleeping tablets. Vitamins may help. Remember that eventually recovery occurs — otherwise it is easy to get despondent. The diagnosis must be made by a doctor, who will consider all the various causes of leg pains before coming to a diagnosis of diabetic neuritis.

A new form of tablet treatment (aldose reductase inhibitors, p.248) for this condition has been introduced recently which is still in the experimental stage but the results so far look quite promising.

35 *I have been a diabetic for many years but my general health is good and I am very stable. During the last year, however, I have developed an extreme soreness on the soles of my feet whenever pressure has been applied, for example when digging with a spade, standing on ladders, walking on hard ground or stones, even when applying the accelerator in the car. If I thump an object with the palm of my hand I suffer the same soreness. The pain is extreme and sometimes lasts for a day or so. Could you tell me if you have heard of this condition in other diabetics and what is the reason for it?*

These symptoms may be due to diabetic neuropathy, a condition which occasionally occurs in long-standing diabetes, due to damage to the nerves. It more often affects the feet than other parts of the body and often produces painful tingling or burning sensations in the feet but perhaps more commonly, numbness. Strict control of the diabetes is important for the prevention and treatment of this complication and it can be made worse by moderate or high alcohol consumption.

36 I am a mild diabetic controlled on diet alone. I suffer from neuritis in my face. My GP says there is no apparent reason for this but I wondered if it had anything to do with my diabetes

There are several types of neuritis affecting the face which have absolutely nothing to do with diabetes. These include shingles (herpes zoster) and Bell's palsy although, of course, both can occur in diabetics. The only forms of diabetic neuritis affecting the face are those that occasionally affect the muscles of the eye leading to double vision and the rare complication known as 'gustatory sweating' where sweating breaks out across the head and scalp at the start of a meal.

37 I have been experiencing a tingling feeling in my fingers. This is worse in the mornings. My doctor says it is neuropathy but knows of no cure for it. Please could you advise me on how my condition could be helped

It is unusual for diabetic neuropathy to affect the hands without it also affecting the feet. If your feet are free from symptoms the most likely cause for the altered sensation in your hands is what is known as the carpal tunnel syndrome which occurs slightly more commonly in diabetics than in non-diabetics. This is due to compression of a nerve in the palm of the hand and can usually be cured by a small operation. It is important to have this investigated at the hospital so bring it to the attention of your doctor when you next visit him, or make a special appointment if your next scheduled visit is a long way off.

38 Is there any treatment for diabetic neuritis apart from trying to keep good diabetic control?

The pain, if there is pain, can be treated with pain-killers, and there are a variety of these so if one particular pain-killer is not effective it is worth trying another one. Occasionally the neuritis will respond to vitamins either by mouth or by injection and lastly there are recent preliminary trials to suggest that a new class of drugs known as aldose reductase inhibitors may prove to be effective for diabetic neuritis. The drugs are still very much at the trial stage and are not generally available yet.

39 *I have recently been told that the tingling sensation in my fingers is due to carpal tunnel syndrome and not neuropathy as was first thought. Can you please explain the difference?*

In the carpal tunnel syndrome (which occurs almost as commonly in non-diabetics as it does in diabetics) the nerves supplying the skin over the fingers, the palm of the hand and some of the muscles in the hand gets compressed at the wrist. Occasionally injections of hydrocortisone or related steroids into the wrist will relieve it and it may require a small operation at the wrist to relieve the tension on the nerve. This usually brings about a dramatic relief of any pain associated with it and a recovery of sensation and muscle strength with time. Diabetic neuropathy more commonly affects the feet than the hands and is usually a painless loss of sensation starting with the tips and moving up the legs or arms. It is only very occasionally painful. This is due to some form of generalized damage to the nerves and is not due to compression of any one nerve. It is much more difficult to treat.

40 *I have been a diabetic for 27 years and have developed a complaint called bowel neuropathy. Please can you explain what this is and what the treatment is?*

Bowel neuropathy is one of the features of autonomic neuropathy which may occur in some long-standing diabetics where there is loss of function of the nerves supplying various organs in the body. In this case, the nerves that regulate the activity of the bowels have been affected. This includes the stomach and the rest of the bowel. The features include indigestion, occasionally vomiting and episodes of alternating constipation and diarrhoea. Occasionally episodes of diarrhoea are preceded by rumblings and gurglings in the stomach and not uncommonly this responds quite well to a short course of antibiotics. Otherwise maintenance of a high-fibre diet is encouraged to prevent constipation. Irritable bowel syndrome can provide symptoms not unlike this and this has nothing to do with diabetes although it commonly occurs in diabetics. If there is ever passage of blood or mucus (slime) within the stool, medical advice should be sought without delay.

41   *The calf muscle in one leg seems to be shrinking. There is no ache and no pain. Is this anything to do with diabetes? I have been taking insulin for 30 years*

You do not mention whether you have noticed any weakness in this leg. Occasionally diabetic neuropathy can affect the nerves which supply the muscles so that the muscle becomes weak and shrinks in size without any accompanying pain or discomfort. It sounds as if this may be your problem.

42   *I suffer from irritation under my skin, my feet, legs, lower body and shoulders. Is this to be expected with diabetes and does it gradually go or is it a permanent symptom?*

The symptoms you describe do not sound at all like a manifestation of diabetic neuropathy and it does not, to me, sound as if it is in any way related to your diabetes.

43   *Please explain a condition called diabetic amyotrophy*

Diabetic amyotrophy is a rare condition causing pain and weakness of the legs and due to damage to certain nerves. It usually occurs when diabetic control is very poor, but occasionally affects people with only slight elevation of the blood sugar. Strict control of the diabetes leads to its improvement but it may take up to 2 years or so for it to settle. The nerves affected are those usually supplying the thigh muscles which often become wasted and get weaker.

Heart and blood vessel disease

44 *I have read that poor circulation of the feet is a problem for diabetics. Is there any way I can improve my circulation?*

Narrowing ('hardening') of the arteries is a normal part of growing older — and the arteries to the feet can be affected by this process, leading to poor circulation in the feet and legs. This occurs in diabetics and non-diabetics, but it is a little commoner in diabetics. We do not fully understand the cause of arterial disease but we do know that smoking makes it worse. So if you are a diabetic and smoke, the risk of bad circulation really does increase. *Stop smoking* and keep active — these are the only known recipes for helping the circulation.

45 *Could you tell me if diabetes is likely to affect the heart of an elderly person? Is such a person likely to develop other ailments such as high blood pressure at this stage?*

Heart disease is only slightly commoner in diabetics than non-diabetics of the same age, but heart disease is of course not uncommon amongst both diabetic and non-diabetics in their seventies. High blood pressure is no commoner amongst diabetics than non-diabetics.

46 *My husband died recently from a heart attack. He had been a diabetic for 12 years controlled on tablets, at about the same time that he developed diabetes he started having angina attacks. I wondered whether these were related and whether poor control had anything to do with his fatal heart attack?*

It sounds as if your husband had trouble with his coronary arteries before be developed diabetes. It is common for people with arterial disease (arteriosclerosis) to develop mild diabetes later in life and it does not sound to me as if his heart attack had anything to do with poor diabetic control.

47 *Is a couple of years of not very good control in a healthy young diabetic likely to have much effect upon the arteries?*

No. It is unlikely to have much of an effect though any period of poor control is not going to do any good either. Our arteries get more rigid and more clogged up as we get older and this process is aggravated by periods of poor diabetic control and smoking.

48 *My left leg was amputated because of diabetic gangrene and I get a lot of pain in my right foot and calf. Could too much insulin be the cause of this pain?*

No. It sounds as if the blood supply to your legs is insufficient and that the pain that you are getting in the foot and calf is a reflection of the poor blood supply which was the reason why you developed gangrene in your left leg.

49 *My husband had a heart attack last year. Nine months later he had part of his leg amputated. We have been told that he could have further problems but have been given no advice. Please give us some information on what we should do to try to avoid this*

It sounds as though your husband has generalized arterial disease (arteriosclerosis) affecting his blood vessels to the heart and to the leg. There are a number of things which you can do which may be of help in preventing further trouble. Firstly, if he smokes, he should stop smoking; secondly his diabetes should be kept as well controlled as possible; thirdly his remaining foot and leg should be kept warm and he should ensure that he has expert foot care either by a chiropodist or by yourself under supervision of a chiropodist or district nurse. If you see any signs of damage to the foot or discoloration then see medical advice at an early stage.

Blood pressure

50 Are diabetics more prone to blood pressure and strokes?

No. Not unless they develop diabetic kidney trouble when the blood pressure can rise as a complication of kidney failure. Strokes are definitely more common in people with high blood pressure.

51 I have been told that my blood pressure is raised as a result of diabetic kidney problems, and because of this it is very important that I take tablets to lower it — why is this?

There is good evidence to show that lowering the blood pressure to normal in patients such as yourself protects the kidneys from further damage and helps delay any further kidney problems.

Smoking

52 We read about Government health warnings concerning the effect of smoking and health. Does this apply to diabetics too?

Indeed it does. It seems that diabetics are particularly at risk as far as smoking and arterial disease (coronaries, strokes and gangrene) but they are no more at risk than non-diabetics as far as lung cancer. There is no reason why any diabetic should smoke.

The mind

53 Can diabetes cause memory loss?

Diabetes does not lead to a poor memory and it is really no excuse for that — except during a hypo!

*54   My 68-year-old mother has been a diabetic for 44 years.
In the past few years her mental state has deteriorated
considerably and she is now difficult to manage. Is this
common for someone who has been on insulin for so
long?*

No, this is not common for someone who has been on insulin
for some time. You fail to mention whether your mother
smokes or not. If she does I suspect that this is much more
likely to be the reason why she has developed cerebral
arteriosclerosis (hardening of the arteries) which may have
contributed to the impairment of her mental functions.

*55   What illnesses or complications could occur in a
diabetic man who had a brain haemorrhage 18 months
ago?*

Brain haemorrhages and strokes are really no more common
in diabetics than in non-diabetics and the management of
somebody who has diabetes and a stroke is really no
different from a non-diabetic with a stroke. The
complications that one would be on the look-out for are
primarily chest infections and pneumonia which need to be
treated early; and also injuries from accidents, if the stroke
sufferer had difficulty in getting about.

*56   Are diabetics more prone to depression, suicide and
other psychiatric illnesses?*

Some evidence suggests that diabetics may be prone to
depression and the suicide rate amongst diabetics is higher
than in the non-diabetic population. Recent studies have
found that the tendency to depression can be relieved in
many cases by more involvement in their own management
and the introduction of home blood glucose monitoring.

*57   I have read that hypos can cause brain damage. Is this
true?*

The strict answer is yes — but only very occasionally. It is
only with hypos associated with long periods of
unconsciousness that brain damage develops, and then it is

extremely unusual. There is no evidence to suggest that the repeated hypos that most insulin-treated diabetics are exposed to do any permanent damage to the brain.

9

Research and the future

Introduction

New developments and improvements in existing treatments can occur only through research. Research is therefore vital to every diabetic. In the UK, the British Diabetic Association spend large sums each year (in 1983–4 £798,000) on research into diabetes, and similar large amounts of money are contributed by the Medical Research Council, the Wellcome Trust and other grant-giving bodies. The more money that is raised for Diabetic research, the greater the benefits to the diabetic community. It costs about £15,000 to support a relatively junior research worker for a year. The discovery of insulin was made by a doctor and a medical student (Banting and Best) doing research together for just one summer (1921). There have been many important but less dramatic discoveries since then, each in some way contributing to our understanding of diabetes and many improving the available treatment.

A cure?

1 Will diabetes ever be cured?

This question cannot be answered — yet. One must always try to take an optimistic view, however, and if diabetes cannot yet be cured it is not for want of research. Not only does the British Diabetic Association have twice yearly meetings to discuss research and progress but there is also an annual European Association for the Study of Diabetes Meeting and an International Diabetes Federation Congress which meets every third year. In addition there are also a great many national organizations which meet regularly. More has been discovered during the past 10 years about the cause of diabetes than ever before and during the same period there have been important advances in treatment. This is, therefore, an exciting period in diabetic research and we may continue to look forward to improvements in our understanding of the disease, even if for the moment cure is a little too much to hope for.

2   *I have a friend who has been treated with insulin for 12 years who recently came off insulin altogether after having had an operation on his adrenal gland. He now tells me that his diabetes has been cured. I thought there was no cure for diabetes*

It sounds as if your friend was one of the few patients in whom the diabetes was secondary to some other condition: in his case, an adrenal tumour which when eventually diagnosed and appropriately treated by operation resulted in a cure in his diabetes. This has been recorded in two forms of adrenal tumour; one is called a phaeochromocytoma, where the tumour produces adrenaline and noradrenaline, both of which inhibit insulin secretion by the pancreas. The other form of adrenal tumour produces an excess of adrenal steroids and cortisone which again produces a form of diabetes which is reversible on removal of the tumour. There are a number of other rare conditions often associated with disturbances of other hormone-producing glands in the body. In these cases cure of diabetes is possible after appropriate therapy of the hormonal disturbance. Unfortunately, less than 5% of all patients with diabetes who have such a hormonal imbalance are amenable to surgery. Specialists are always on the look-out for these causes since the benefits from operation are so tremendous.

3 Will it ever be possible to prevent diabetes with a vaccine?

There is some evidence to suggest that certain virus infections can cause diabetes but we are not clear what proportion of newly diagnosed diabetes are caused by a virus infection; it is probably very low. If a virus was isolated which caused diabetes, then it should be possible to produce a vaccine which could be given to children like polio vaccine, to prevent them from developing diabetes later on in life. At present this possibility seems rather remote.

4 My son's diabetes has recently gone into remission following 3 months treatment with insulin. I have been told that this is the 'honeymoon period' and is likely to last only a few weeks or a few months. Is there any way this honeymoon period can be extended and turned into a cure?

Some research work has been done in this area using anti-viral agents and drugs that interfere with the body's immune responses. The results so far do not show any positive benefit from the anti-viral preparations but do suggest that the immunosuppressive therapy may prolong the 'honeymoon period' in some patients. Unfortunately this form of therapy itself is not without risks and it certainly cannot be recommended until the results of full scientific trials have been reported.

5 I gather that it is possible to identify people within a family who are at high risk of developing diabetes by looking at special blood tests. This sounds like an exciting development; presumably children who have inherited a susceptibility to diabetes will be those most in need of vaccination should a vaccine become available

Yes, you are right. Studies of the so-called HLA tissue antigens in families where there appears to be a lot of diabetes indicates that certain patterns of inherited antigens carry with them the susceptibility to diabetes, and using these markers it should be possible to identify the children who are likely to benefit most from a vaccine or an effective form of preventative treatment should one become available. It will be in these individuals that the first clinical trials will need to be done.

Transplantation

6　*I would like to volunteer to have a pancreas transplant. Is there someone I must apply to? How successful have these operations been?*

Pancreatic transplantation is still in the experimental stages and it will be difficult to find anyone who will accept you as a volunteer. Technically, pancreatic transplants are more difficult than even liver, kidney or heart transplants. The pancreas is delicate and, as the seat of many digestive juices, has a tendency to digest itself if damaged even slightly. The duct or passageway through which these juices pass is narrow, and has to be joined up to the intestines in a very intricate way so that the enzymes do not leak. Even if everything goes well, technically the body will still react against the transplant so several immunosuppressant drugs have to be given. Some of these (particularly steroids) given in high doses to suppress rejection of the transplant tend to cause diabetes or make existing diabetes worse! Some hospitals have carried out this operation successfully. At the moment, these centres do the operation only if another transplant (usually a kidney) is also necessary, since only a proportion of pancreatic transplants work. Pancreatic transplants have been done in London, Birmingham and Cambridge, but none of these centres are asking for volunteers yet.

7　*Are there any hospitals that carry out transplants of the islets of Langerhans? Would I be able to donate my cells to my diabetic daughter?*

No, there are no hospitals carrying out such transplants yet, and it would not be possible for you to donate your pancreatic islet cells to your daughter. The question you raise, however, is an important one because experiments carried out in animals show that it is technically possible to isolate the islets of Langerhans of a non-diabetic animal and transplant them into a diabetic animal and cure the diabetes. There are two main steps to be overcome before this technique is available for humans. Firstly, one has to find a way of culturing and growing the islet cells in a laboratory so that one can produce enough of them to transplant into a diabetic to produce enough insulin to cure the condition. Secondly, we have to get over the problems of transplantation of tissues from one individual to another: we have to prevent rejection of the transplant. Traditionally in kidney and other organ transplants this is done by giving large doses of steroids and immunosuppressive drugs. This form of treatment unfortunately has its own risks. These risks may be justifiable when the alternative is death through renal failure or heart failure. However, in the diabetic there is an effective form of treatment in the form of insulin injections which carries with it in the long term much less hazard to health than immunosuppressive therapy.

It is therefore quite clear at present that until there has been a major breakthrough in transplantation of tissues from one individual to another, the hazards of long-term immunosuppressive therapy for a diabetic receiving either a pancreas transplant or an islet transplant are far greater than having diabetes treated with insulin. There are no tangible benefits yet for this form of therapy as a primary form of treatment for diabetes. This does not mean that the problems are insuperable but that much research remains to be done before the problems are overcome.

Insulin pumps and artificial pancreas

8 *I recently read about a device called a 'glucose sensor' which can control the insulin administered to diabetic animals. Will this ever be used on humans, and if so what can we expect from it?*

The research into the development of a small electronic device which could be implanted under the skin and which

could continuously monitor the level of glucose in the blood
has been going on in the United States, the United Kingdom
and several countries for many years. The technical
problems of such a device are, however, considerable, and it
seems unlikely to be of use in diabetics at least for some
considerable time. Not only are there technical problems in
achieving an accurate reflection of blood glucose level by
such a subcutaneous implanted glucose sensor, but the
further problem of 'hooking it up' to a supply of insulin to be
released according to the demand is formidable. However, it
may be that these problems may one day be resolved and one
might then hope that better control of diabetes might be
achieved than can be achieved by the current methods.
There is, however, a long way to go yet.

9   *I have heard about the artificial pancreas or 'Biostator'.*
Apparently this machine is capable of maintaining a
diabetic's blood sugar at absolutely normal values,
irrespective of what they eat. Is this true? If so, why is it
not widely available?

There are several versions of what you describe, namely an
'artificial pancreas', which measures the glucose concentration in the bloodstream continuously and infuses insulin in
sufficient quantities to keep the blood glucose normal.
Unfortunately these machines are technically very complex,
bulky and extremely expensive. Their major value is for
research purposes since they are quite unsuitable at present
as devices for long-term control. Their use has, however,
taught us a lot about the needs of such a device in the future,
when it can be scaled down to something the same size as a
cardiac pacemaker. There is a great deal of research going
on amongst several bio-engineering groups to achieve this
aim but it is still likely to be several years before the first of
several machines become available for research studies and
it will be a long time before suitably reliable machines are
available for daily treatment. Even when the technical
problems have been resolved and it has been miniaturized to
an acceptable size for implantation the costs are likely to be a
limiting factor governing availability. The currently

available, rather crude machines weigh in excess of 20 kg (44 lb) and cost thousands of pounds. There is much work to be done before this becomes a viable form of treatment.

10   What are the likely developments with insulin pumps within the next 5 years?

'Open loop' insulin pumps that infuse insulin at a programmed rate without any link to a blood glucose sensing device are becoming increasingly available in smaller, more compact and more sophisticated forms. Unfortunately, the price also tends to increase which limits their availability. It is probable that over the next 5 years these prices will fall as the sophisticated electronic technology required becomes cheaper. As discussed in Chapter 2 (p.31), these pumps are really only suitable for a proportion of insulin-treated patients in their current form and the major breakthrough will occur when there has been a reliable link built between the glucose sensor and the insulin infusion pump, producing a 'true' artificial pancreas.

New insulins and oral insulins

11   What advances can we expect in the development of new insulin?

Over the last 10 years we have gone through a stage of producing increasingly purer insulins with patterns of absorption varying from the very quick acting to the very long acting formulations. Most recently we have had available the human insulin preparations produced synthetically and it is likely that the price of these insulins will fall as supplies become more plentiful. What we are looking for next is variation in the structure or formulations of the insulins which will improve the reliability of the absorption from the site in which they are injected to eliminate the variations that occur daily with current insulin preparations. We are also looking for variations in the structure of the insulin which will 'target' the insulin more directly on the liver, the major organ responsible for glucose production in the body. Normally insulin is produced by the pancreas and goes directly to the liver. Unfortunately, in insulin-treated patients the insulin which is injected only reaches the liver after it has been through all the other tissues in the body. It should be possible to modify the structure in such a way that it can be targetted at the liver and in that way perhaps turn out to be a more effective and easier way of controlling blood glucose level in diabetics.

12 *I have heard that it is possible to get away from insulin injections by either putting drops up the nose or by producing some form of insulin which is active when taken by mouth. Are these claims true and are we going to be able to get away from insulin injections in the future?*

There is no doubt that a small proportion of insulin put up the nose is absorbed through the membranes into the bloodstream and can lower the blood sugar. Unfortunately only a small percentage of that which is put into the nose is ever absorbed and it is an inefficient and therefore expensive way of administering insulin. Because the absorption is rather erratic it also produces rather erratic changes in blood glucose. Experiments have been done with insulin suppositories showing that they too can lower the blood sugar without the need for injection but again the absorption is only incomplete and the response erratic. It is possible that new methods will be found for increasing the absorption from these two sites and making this a possible alternative mode of insulin administration. Regarding oral insulins, it is possible to prevent the stomach digesting the insulin by incorporating it into a fat droplet (liposome). This enables it to be absorbed from the gut without being broken down by the digestive juices. Unfortunately, the absorption is erratic and the whole lipid droplet with the insulin is absorbed, the insulin remaining inactive until it is released from the droplet. So far technical problems with this have not been solved despite a great deal of research and, at present, it seems unlikely that effective oral insulins will be developed in the foreseeable future.

New technology

13   What benefits to diabetics are going to come from the computer and micro-electronic revolution?

You will have already seen some of the benefits in the blood glucose monitoring devices. All of the modern insulin pumps rely heavily on micro-chips to control the rate of infusion and its programming. We are beginning to see micro-computer programmes which help store and analyse home blood glucose monitoring records and it should be possible soon to simulate the blood glucose response to different insulin injections and in this way produce means of exploring the effect of different types and doses of insulin and simulating the body's response. We are also going to experience the use of computers as a way of teaching patients about diabetes and its management as well as a way of testing patients about their knowledge of diabetes. Micro-computers are being used to help record and analyse records from the diabetic clinic as well as to help to plan and organize monitoring of diabetic care and this is quite likely to lead to an improvement in the efficiency of the organization of the diabetic clinics as it has done to the organizing of airline tickets and flights. There are early experiments going on in the use of so-called 'expert systems' to transfer the expert knowledge of specialists to general practitioners to facilitate their management of diabetic patients within the general practice environment without the need for patients to attend hospital diabetic clinics so often. It is not unreasonable to expect that the micro-electronic revolution will produce a lot of benefits to the diabetic over the next 10 years.

10

Self-help groups

Introduction

This section is a description of various organizations that have grown up to help diabetics help themselves. It is a straight description of what is available and is not written in the style of question and answer.

People react in different ways to the shock of diabetes; some try to become recluses and hide, while others set out to try to solve all the problems of mankind (including diabetes) in a few weeks. Whatever your reaction, you should make contact with your local Diabetic Association. You will come across people who are *living* with diabetes and who have learnt to cope with many of the daily problems. These people should provide an extra dimension to the information you have been given by the doctors, nurses and dietitians at the clinic.

The British Diabetic Association (BDA)

This was founded in 1934 by two diabetics, H G Wells the author and R D Lawrence, who was a doctor based at the diabetic clinic of King's College Hospital, London. In a letter to *The Times*, dated January 1933, they announced their intention to set up an 'Association open to all diabetics, rich or poor, for mutual aid and assistance, and to promote the study, the diffusion of knowledge, and the proper treatment of diabetes in this country.' They proposed that diabetics, members of the general public interested in diabetes and doctors and nurses should be persuaded to join the projected Association. Fifty years later, the British Diabetic Association is a credit to its founders. It has 100,000 members, 50 permanent administrative staff and an annual budget of £2.1 million. Like any large organization, the BDA has its faults, but it keeps a balance of interest between diabetics and those who are there to help diabetics. In many countries there are separate organizations for patients and for professionals but the BDA draws its strength from the fact that both interest groups are united in the same society.

The BDA is the biggest provider in the UK of funds for diabetic research and the target for 1984, its fiftieth jubilee year, was to raise one million pounds for research into all aspects of diabetes.

The BDA also provides help and advice to diabetics and their families. It publishes an excellent news magazine, called *Balance*, which appears every other month. The BDA also produces a handbook, leaflets and videotapes for teaching purposes.

BDA Camps

The first BDA holiday for children took place in 1935, and 'the camps' have grown into a large enterprise. There are now about 30 camps each year catering for up to a 1000 diabetic children, aged 7–16 years. These educational holidays are organized centrally by the Youth Department and they aim to give the children a good time, to teach them more about their diabetes and to provide a well-earned break for their parents. Equally important is the opportunity they give children to meet other diabetics and to become more independent of their parents.

The Youth Department also organizes weekends for parents of children with diabetes. These cater for up to 30 family groups. The children are entertained by trained helpers while the parents receive talks from specialist doctors, nurses and dietitians. There are also talks from parents who have lived with diabetic children for many years and from young adults who have made a success of their lives, despite the problem of diabetes. These parent/child weekends are designed to encourage an informal atmosphere.

Local BDA Branches

There are over 200 branches throughout the country. These are run entirely by volunteers and because of their commitment large sums of money are raised for diabetic research. The BDA branches also aim to increase public awareness of diabetes and arrange meetings for local diabetics and their families.

Parents' Groups

Parents of young diabetic children often feel that they have special needs — and can offer particular help to other parents in the same boat. Nearly a hundred parents' groups exist throughout the UK and they have added a sense of urgency to the main aim of the BDA; namely the defeat of diabetes. In addition to self-help, the parents' groups also raise money for research.

National Diabetes Foundation (NDF)

The NDF was founded in 1982 and has made ground in several parts of the country. It is a sister organization of the Juvenile Diabetes Federation (JDF) which grew up in America in the 1970s as a breakaway from the American Diabetes Association. The JDF is primarily concerned with raising funds for research in order to find a cure for diabetes. If we go back to the original aims of the BDA ('for mutual aid and assistance, and to promote the study and proper treatment of diabetes in this country'), any group that shares these aims must be a good thing. Perhaps the NDF has the negative effect of fragmenting the effort of the BDA.

The Sheffield Pump Club

Dr John Ward at the Royal Hallamshire Hospital in Sheffield is carrying out a large project (with financial support from the BDA) to discover how ordinary diabetics cope with an insulin pump for controlling their blood sugar. The Pump Club is an informal self-help group of those taking part in the survey.

Firbush — Young Diabetic Leaders

This is a special kind of BDA camp organized by Professor Farquar of Edinburgh University. Jim Farquar is a paediatrician who has a special interest in helping young adults with diabetes. He has known for a long time that the best teacher for a young diabetic is another young diabetic. In 1983 he took 20 diabetics from all parts of the UK to Firbush, a custom-built adventure centre on the banks of Loch Tay. As well as canoeing, sailing, cycling and climbing the young people worked in groups to try to identify the problems of the young diabetic and to decide how they could help other young people in their own locality. The Firbush experiment is being repeated annually and is the beginning of a national self-help movement for young diabetics.

11

Emergencies

Introduction

This section of the book is for quick reference if things are
going badly wrong. Firstly there is vital information for the
diabetic himself and then some simple rules for relatives and
friends. They are designed to be consulted in an emergency,
though it would be worth checking through them *before* you
reach crisis point. It seems a pity to end this book in such a
negative way by telling you what to do in a crisis. We hope
that by keeping your diabetes well controlled you will avoid
these serious situations.

What every diabetic on insulin must know

1 **NEVER** stop insulin if you feel ill or sick. Check your
   blood sugar — you may need extra insulin even though
   you are not eating very much.
2 If you are being sick, try to keep up a good fluid intake (at
   least 4 pints a day). If you are vomiting and unable to
   keep down fluids, you probably need to go to hospital for
   an intravenous drip.
3 ALWAYS CARRY SUGAR on your person. NEVER risk
   driving if your blood sugar could be low. Diabetics *DO*

lose their driving licences if found at the wheel when hypo.

4   Physical exercise and alcohol are both likely to bring on a hypo.

What other people must know about diabetes

1   **NEVER** stop insulin in case of sickness (no apologies for repeating this).

2   Repeated vomiting, drowsiness and laboured breathing are bad signs in a diabetic. They suggest impending coma and can be treated ONLY in hospital.

3   A diabetic who is hypo may not be in full command of his senses and may take a lot of persuasion to have some sugar. Jam or a sugary drink (Lucozade) may be easier to get down than dextrose tablets.

4   **NEVER** let a diabetic drive if you suspect he is hypo. It could be fatal.

Foods to eat in an emergency or when feeling unwell

Each of the following contains *10 g* carbohydrate:

100 ml pure fruit juice
100 ml Coca Cola (*Not* Diet Coke)
60 ml Lucozade
Small scoop ice cream
2 sugar cubes or 2 teaspoons of sugar
1 jelly cube or 2 heaped tablespoons of made up jelly
$\frac{1}{3}$ pint of milk
Egg flip made with $\frac{1}{3}$ pint of milk, 1 egg and a drop of vanilla essence
2 cream crackers
1 packet of crisps
1 natural yoghurt
1 apple or pear or orange
1 small banana
3 Dextrosol tablets.

If you are feeling unwell, eating solid food may not be possible and you may need to rely on sweet fluids to provide the necessary carbohydrate. Liquids such as cold, defizzed Coca-Cola or Lucozade are useful if you feel sick. Do not worry about eating the exact amount of carbohydrate at the correct time but take small amounts often.

If you continue to vomit, **SEEK MEDICAL ADVICE.**

Foods suitable as extra carbohydrate when exercising

Each snack contains *20 g* carbohydrate:

    1 glass Coca-Cola (220 ml)
    1 mini-size Mars bar or Milky Way
    4 squares chocolate
    2 big digestive biscuits
    2 small packets (40 g) of nuts and raisins.

Signs and symptoms of hypoglycaemia and hyperglycaemia

Hypoglycaemia = LOW blood sugar. Also called a 'hypo', a reaction or an insulin reaction.
    Fast onset.

        Tingling of the lips and tongue
        Weakness
        Tiredness
        Sleepiness
        Trembling
        Hunger
        Blurred vision
        Palpitation
        Nausea
        Headache
        Sweating
        Mental confusion
        Pallor
        Slurred speech
        Bad temper

Change in behaviour
Lack of concentration
Unconsciousness (hypoglycaemic or insulin coma).

Hyperglycaemia = HIGH blood sugar.
  Slow onset (usually more than 24 hours).

Thirst
Excess urine
Nausea
Abdominal pain
Vomiting
Drowsiness
Rapid breathing
Flushed, dry skin
Unconsciousness (hyperglycaemic or diabetic coma).

Appendix 1

Glossary of terms

Acesulfane-K   A low-calorie 'intense' sweetener.

Acetone   A chemical substance formed when the body uses body fat for energy. The presence of acetone in the urine means that insufficient insulin is being taken.

Adrenaline   A hormone produced by the adrenal glands which prepares the body for action ('flight or fight') and also causes an increase in blood glucose level. It is produced by the body when the blood glucose falls too low.

Albumin   A protein present in most animal tissues. The presence of albumin in the urine may denote a kidney or bladder infection or early kidney damage.

Aldose reductase inhibitor   A drug which blocks the enzyme aldose reductase, reducing the accumulation of sorbitol in tissues. Its use is being explored in the treatment and prevention of diabetic complications. So far there is no definite proof that it is effective.

Alpha cell   The cell that produces glucagon — found in the islets of Langerhans in the pancreas.

Arteriosclerosis   Hardening of the arteries. A loss of elasticity in the walls of the arteries due to thickening and calcification. It occurs with advancing years in those with or without diabetes. This may affect the heart, causing thrombosis, or it may affect the circulation particularly of the legs and feet.

Aspartame   A low-calorie 'intense' sweetener. Brand name 'Nutra-Sweet'.

Autonomic neuropathy   Damage to the system of nerves which regulate many automatic functions of the body such as stomach emptying, sexual function (potency) and blood pressure control.

Balanitis   Inflammation of the end of the penis, usually caused by the presence of sugar in the urine.

Beta blockers   Drugs which block the effect of stress hormones on the cardiovascular system. They are often used to treat angina and to lower blood pressure. They may also change the warning signs of hypoglycaemia.

Beta cell   The cell which produces insulin — found in the islets of Langerhans in the pancreas.

Biguanides   A group of anti-diabetes tablets which lower blood glucose levels. They work by increasing the uptake of glucose by muscle, by reducing the absorption of glucose by the intestine and by reducing the amount of glucose produced by the liver. The most commonly used preparation is metformin.

Blood glucose monitoring   A system of measuring blood glucose levels at home using special reagent sticks or a special meter.

Bran   The indigestible husk of the wheat grain which is a high source of fibre or roughage.

Brittle diabetes   A term used to refer to diabetes which is very unstable with swings from very low to very high blood glucose levels.

Calories   The units in which energy or heat are measured. The energy value of food is measured in calories.

Carbohydrates   A class of food which comprises starches and sugars and is most readily available by the body for energy. They are found mainly in plant foods. Examples are rice, bread, potatoes, pasta, dried beans.

Cataract   Opacity of the lens of the eye which obscures vision. It may be removed surgically.

Control   Usually refers to blood glucose control. The aim of good control is to achieve normal blood glucose levels (3–7 mmol/l).

Cystitis   Inflammation of the bladder causing frequency of passing urine and a burning sensation when passing urine.

Diabetic amyotrophy A rare condition causing pain and/or weakness of the legs due to the damage to certain nerves.

Diabetic coma An extreme form of hyperglycaemia, usually with ketoacidosis associated with unconsciousness.

Diuretic An agent which increases the flow of urine, usually called 'water tablets'.

'Double voided' Passing one sample of urine and discarding it before passing a second sample within an hour, for the purpose of urine testing.

Epidural Usually referring to the type of anaesthetic that is used commonly in obstetrics. Anaesthetic solution is injected through the spinal canal to numb the lower part of the body.

Exchanges Portions of carbohydrate foods in the diabetic diet which can be exchanged for one another. 1 exchange = 10 grams carbohydrate.

Fibre The part of plant material which resists digestion and gives bulk to the diet. Also known as roughage.

Free foods Foods which contain so little carbohydrate (or fat) that diabetics may have liberal helpings without counting them in their diet. Examples include cabbage, rhubarb, lettuce, cauliflower, tea or coffee without milk.

Fructose A type of sugar found naturally in fruit and honey. Since it does not require insulin for its metabolism, is often used as a sweetener in diabetic foods.

Gangrene Death of a part of the body due to a very poor blood supply. A combination of neuropathy and arteriosclerosis may result in infection of unrecognized injuries to the feet. If neglected this infection may spread, causing further destruction.

Gestational diabetes Occurs in women who become diabetic during pregnancy and who then return to normal after their babies are born.

Glaucoma A disease of the eye causing increased pressure inside the eyeball.

Glucagon A hormone produced by the alpha cells in the pancreas which causes a rise in blood glucose by freeing glycogen from the liver. It is available in injection form and can be used to treat a severe hypo.

Glucose   A form of sugar made by digestion of carbohydrates. It is absorbed into the bloodstream where it circulates and is used for energy.

Glucose tolerance test   A test used in the diagnosis of diabetes mellitus. The glucose in the blood is measured at intervals before and after the person has drunk a large amount of glucose whilst fasting.

Glycogen   The form in which carbohydrate is stored in the liver. It is often known as animal starch.

Glycosuria   The presence of glucose in the urine.

Guar   A high source of dietary fibre obtainable from the cluster bean.

Haemoglobin A$_1$ The part of the haemoglobin or colouring matter of the red blood cell which has glucose attached to it. It is a useful test of diabetic control as the amount of haemoglobin A$_1$ in the blood depends on how high the blood glucose levels have been for the previous month or two.

'Honeymoon period'   The time when the dose of insulin drops shortly after starting insulin treatment. It is the result of partial recovery of insulin secretion by the pancreas. Usually the honeymoon period only lasts for a short time.

Hormone   A substance which is generated in one gland or organ and is carried by the blood to another part of the body to stimulate another organ into activity.

Hydramnios   An excessive amount of amniotic fluid, i.e. the fluid surrounding the fetus.

Hyperglycaemia   High blood glucose or blood sugar (above 10 mmol/l).

Hypoglycaemia   Low blood glucose or blood sugar (below 2.5 mmol/l).

Insulin   A hormone produced by the beta cells of the pancreas and responsible for the control of blood glucose. Insulin can only be given by injection because the digestive juices destroy its action if it is taken by mouth.

Insulin coma   The extreme form of hypoglycaemia associated with unconsciousness and sometimes convulsions.

Insulin dependent diabetes (IDD)   The type of diabetes which cannot be treated without insulin. It is most common in younger people and is also called type I diabetes or juvenile-onset diabetes.

Insulin reaction Another name for hypoglycaemia or a 'hypo'. In America it is called an 'insulin shock' or 'shock'.

Intradermal Meaning 'into the skin'. Usually refers to an injection given into the most superficial layer of the skin. Insulin must not be given in this way as it is painful and will not be absorbed properly.

Intramuscular A deep injection into the muscle.

Joules A unit of work or energy used in the metric system. There are about 4.18 joules in each calorie. Some dietitians now calculate food energy in joules.

Juvenile-onset diabetes An outdated name for insulin-dependent diabetes, so called because most patients receiving insulin develop diabetes under the age of 40. The term is no longer used because insulin-dependent diabetes can occur at any age.

Ketoacidosis A serious condition due to lack of insulin which results in body fat being used up to form ketones and acids. It is characterized by high blood glucose levels, ketones in the urine, vomiting, drowsiness, heavy laboured breathing and a smell of acetone on the breath.

Ketones Acid substances formed when body fat is used up to provide energy.

Ketonuria The presence of acetone and other ketones in the urine. They can be detected by testing with a special testing stick (Ketostix) or tablet (Acetest). The presence of ketones is due to lack of insulin or periods of starvation.

Laser treatment A process in which laser beams are used to treat a damaged retina (back of the eye) (see photocoagulation).

Lipoatrophy The loss of fat from injection sites. It used to occur before the use of highly purified insulins.

Lipohypertrophy An excessive accummulation of fat, usually caused by using the same areas for injection too frequently.

Maturity onset Another term for non-insulin dependent diabetes most commonly occurring in people who are middle aged and overweight. Also called type II diabetes.

Metabolism The process by which the body turns food into energy.

Microaneurysms Small red dots on the retina at the back of the eye which are one of the earliest signs of diabetic retinopathy. They represent areas of weakness of the very small blood vessels in the eye.

Millimoles New units for measuring the concentration of glucose and other substances in the blood. Blood glucose is measured in millimoles per litre (mmol/l). It has replaced milligrammes per decilitre (mg/dl or mg%) as a unit of measurement and which is still used in other countries. 1 mmol/l = 18 mg/dl.

Nephropathy Kidney damage. In the first instance this makes the kidney more leaky so that albumin appears in the urine. At a later stage it may affect the function of the kidney and in severe cases lead to kidney failure.

Neuropathy Damage to the nerves. This may be peripheral or automatic (see peripheral neuropathy or autonomic neuropathy). It can occur with diabetes especially when poorly controlled, but also has other causes.

Non-insulin dependent diabetic (NIDD) The type of diabetes which occurs in older people who are often overweight. These people do not always need insulin treatment and usually can be successfully controlled with diet alone or diet and tablets. Also known as type II or maturity onset diabetes.

Pancreas The gland lying behind the stomach which as well as secreting a digestive fluid (pancreatic juice) also produces the hormone, insulin.

Peripheral neuropathy Damage to the nerves supplying muscles and skin. This can result in diminished sensation, particularly in the feet and legs, and in muscle weakness.

Photocoagulation A process of treating diabetic retinopathy with light beams, either laser beams or 'xenon arc'. This technique focusses a beam of light on a very tiny area of the retina. This beam is so intense that it causes a small burn, which may close off a leaking blood vessel or destroy weak blood vessels which are likely to bleed.

Protein One of the classes of food that is necessary for growth and repair of tissues. It is found in fish, meat, eggs, milk and pulses (dried peas and beans). It can also refer to albumin when found in the urine.

Proteinuria Protein or albumin in the urine (see albumin).

Pruritus vulvae Irritation of the vulva. This is caused by an infection that occurs because of an excess of sugar in the urine and is often an early sign of diabetes in the older diabetic. It clears up when the blood glucose levels return to normal and the sugar disappears from the urine.

Polydipsia Being excessively thirsty and drinking too much. Also a symptom of untreated diabetes.

Polyuria The passing of large quantities of urine due to excess glucose from the bloodstream. It is a symptom of untreated diabetes.

Pyelonephritis Inflammation and infection of the kidney.

Renal threshold The level of glucose in the blood above which it will begin to spill into the urine. The usual renal threshold for glucose in about 10 mmol/l, i.e. when the blood glucose rises above 10 mmol/l, glucose appears in the urine.

Retina The light-sensitive coat at the back of the eye.

Retinopathy Damage to the retina.

Saccharine A synthetic sweetener which is calorie free.

Sorbitol A chemical related to sugar and alcohol which is used as a sweetening agent. It has no significant effect upon the blood sugar level but has the same number of calories as ordinary sugar so should not be used by those who need to lose weight. It is poorly absorbed and may have a laxative effect.

Subcutaneous injection An injection beneath the skin into the layer of fat which lies between the skin and muscle.

Sucrose A sugar (containing glucose and fructose in combination) derived from sugar cane or sugar beet (i.e. ordinary table sugar). It has a high carbohydrate and calorie content.

Sulphonylureas Antidiabetes tablets which lower the blood glucose by stimulating the pancreas to produce more insulin. Commonly used sulphonylureas are glibenclamide, chlorpropamide and tolbutamide.

Toxaemia Poisoning of the blood by the absorption of toxins. Usually refers to the toxaemia of pregnancy which is characterized by high blood pressure, proteinuria and ankle swelling.

U 100 insulin   The standard strength of insulin in the UK, USA, Canada, Australia and New Zealand. It refers to 100 units of insulin per millilitre.

'Visual acuity'   Acuteness of vision. Measured by reading letters on a sight testing chart (Snellen chart).

Appendix 2

Useful addresses

Ames Division
Miles Laboratories Ltd
Stoke Court
Stoke Poges
Slough
Berkshire SL2 4LY
Tel: 02814 5151

Becton Dickinson UK Ltd
Between Towns Road
Cowley
Oxford OX4 3LY
Tel: 0865 777722

Bochringer Corporation Ltd
Boehringer Mannheim House
Bell Lane
Lewes
East Sussex BN7 1LG
Tel: 07916 71611

Britannia Pharmaceuticals Ltd
Hamilton House
87–89 Bell Street
Reigate
Surrey RH2 7YZ
Tel: 07372 22256

British Diabetic Association
10 Queen Anne Street
London W1M 0BD
Tel: 01 323 1531

Clinitron Bio-Medical
    Instruments
Clinitron House
Savile Bridge
Savile Road
Dewsbury
West Yorkshire WF12 9AF
Tel: 0924 461556

Eli Lilly & Co. Ltd
Kingsclere Road
Basingstoke
Hants RG21 2XA
Tel: 0256 473241

Genetics International (UK)
    Inc.
11 Nuffield Way
Abingdon
Oxon OX14 1RL
Tel: 0235 34242

Graseby Medical
Units 3–4 Odhams Trading
  Estate
St Albans Road
Watford
Herts WD2 5JX
Tel: 0923 44464

Hypoguard Ltd
Dock Lane
Melton
Woodbridge
Suffolk IP12 1PE
Tel: 03943 7333/4

Large Type Books for
  Partially Sighted
Ulverscroft Books
The Green
Bradgate Road
Ansley
Leicester LE7 7FW
Tel: 053 721 4325

Mariner Medical Ltd
Diabetic Consumer Unit
Mariner House
116 Windmill Street
Gravesend
Kent DA12 1BL
Tel: 0474 23456
(Suppliers of Monoject
  Equipment)

MCP Pharmaceuticals Ltd
Simpson Parkway
Kirkton Campus
Livingston
West Lothian
Tel: 0506 412512

Medic Alert Foundation
11/13 Clifton Terrace
London N4 3JP
Tel: 01 263 8596

Medistron Ltd
6 Lawson-Hunt Industrial
  Park
Broadbridge Heath
West Sussex RH12 3JR
Tel: 0403 64823

Monoject Products
Sherwood Medical Industries
  Ltd
London Road
County Oak
Crawley
West Sussex RH10 2TL
Tel: 0293 34501

Nordisk UK
Highview House
Tattenham Crescent
Epsom Downs
Epsom
Surrey KT18 5OJ
Tel: 073 73 60621

Novo Laboratories Ltd
Ringway House
Bell Road
Daneshill East
Basingstoke
Hampshire RG24 0QN
Tel: 0256 55055

Owen Mumford Ltd Medical
  Shop
Brook Hill
Woodstock
Oxon OX7 1TU
Tel: 0993 812862

Palmer Injector Ltd
11 George Square
Glasgow G2 1EA
Tel: 041 248 6413

Parisian Medical and Scientific
18 the Osiers Estate
Osiers Road
London SW18 1NL
Tel: 01 871 1344

Rand Rocket
ABCare House
Walsworth Road
Hitchin
Herts SG4 9SX
Tel: 0462 58871

The Royal National Institute
   for the Blind
224 Great Portland Street
London W1
Tel: 01 388 1266

Rybar Laboratories Ltd
29 Hill Avenue
Amersham
Bucks HP6 5BX
Tel: 02403 22741

SOS/Talisman
Golden Key Co.
9–11 High Street
Sheerness
Kent

Index

Numbers in italics refer to question numbers not page references